Table of Contents

Skin Care and Beauty Recipes
  - Nourishing Facial Serum
  - Acne-Blasting Spot Treatment
  - Radiant Hair Mask

Household Cleaning Recipes
  - Natural All-Purpose Cleaner
  - Sparkling Dishwasher Tabs
  - Fresh Linen Spray

Aromatic Remedies
  - Soothing Muscle Salve
  - Earache Relief Oil
  - Sinus Congestion Inhalation Blend

Favorite Recipes
  - Homemade Makeup Remover
  - Lavender and Rose Water Toner
  - Calming Body Butter
  - Body Butter Lotion
  - Face Wash
  - Homemade Body Wash
  - Coconut Lavender Shampoo
  - Eye Cream
  - Anti-aging Serum
  - Morning Eye Cream
  - Shaving Cream
  - Beard Oil
  - Allergy & Cold Remedy
  - Laundry Soap

∞ ∞ ∞

Introduction: Aromatherapy & Essential Oils

Welcome to "Aromatherapy & Essential Oils" in this beautifully curated collection of recipes, providing you with the tools to harness the incredible power of essential oils. Our recipes have been crafted to create a harmonious environment for yourself and your loved ones. Whether seeking relaxation, stress relief, a burst of energy, or motivation, this recipe book will be your trusted companion on your aromatic journey.

Gone are the days of relying on store-bought air fresheners and chemical-filled products. It's time to embrace the natural wonders of the aromatic world. With the recipes in this book, you will create your own all-natural, chemical-free blends that promote wellness, enhancing the ambiance of the world around you.

Immerse yourself in the exquisite scents and therapeutic benefits of essential oils. Indulge in the calming properties of lavender, peppermint's uplifting nature, or chamomile's soothing effects. Mix and match to find the perfect blend that suits your needs and preferences.

By using our recipes, you are not only creating a healthy and harmonious environment but also minimizing your exposure to harmful chemicals. Embrace the power of nature and let it fill your home with delightful aromas that will uplift your spirits and rejuvenate your mind.

So, say goodbye to synthetic fragrances and hello to the wonders of essential oils. Discover the art of aromatherapy and unlock the numerous benefits it has to offer. Let "Aromatherapy Delights: Essential Oils Recipe Book" guide you and embark on a journey of self-care and well-being.

∞ ∞ ∞

History of Essential Oils

Tracing back to ancient civilizations, essential oils are valued for their medicinal, aromatic, and spiritual properties. In ancient Egypt, essential oils were extracted from plants like frankincense and myrrh and were an integral part of religious ceremonies and the embalming process for mummification. Similarly, ancient Indian Ayurvedic medicine incorporated essential oils for their therapeutic benefits, including treating various ailments and promoting overall wellness. Essential oils also played a significant role in traditional Chinese medicine, used for healing properties and to balance the body's energy.

As the centuries passed, essential oils have continued to have unique scents and healing attributes. They were transported and traded along the Silk Road, leading to their introduction and popularity in Europe during the Renaissance period. Essential oils are used in perfumes, natural remedies, and flavorings in food and beverages.

In the present day, essential oils have experienced a resurgence in popularity due to their natural health benefits and role in aromatherapy. They are extracted through various methods, such as steam distillation or cold pressing, preserving their aromatic and therapeutic qualities. Essential oils can be found in products, including cosmetics, fragrances, cleaning supplies, and culinary preparations, adding depth and flavor to dishes.

The demand for pure and high-quality essential oils continues to grow as more people recognize their potential to enhance well-being and promote a holistic approach to health.

Whether essential oils are to relax and destress, uplift mood, boost immunity, or relieve various discomforts, they have become part of many self-care routines. With their rich history and versatile uses, essential oils offer a sensory journey into the past while supporting overall wellness in the present.

Understanding Essential Oils

Essential oils have a long history of use in various cultural practices worldwide. These oils derive from incredibly concentrated plants, capturing the aromatic scents and flavors. Making them powerful tools for promoting overall wellness and improving physical and emotional well-being. Many people turn to essential oils for their purported health benefits, which include stress relief, improved sleep, and enhanced immune function.

However, it is crucial to exercise caution when using essential oils. With proper knowledge and guidance will decrease adverse effects and harm. To have an understanding of essential oils, knowing their extraction methods is helpful. Different plants have different requirement methods, such as steam distillation or cold pressing, to extract their oils effectively.

Additionally, proper dilution techniques are crucial. Essential oils are highly concentrated and should not be applied directly to the skin or ingested before dilution. Mixing them with carrier oils such as coconut or almond oils will ensure proper use and prevent skin irritation or other reactions.

Furthermore, it is essential to consider potential interactions with medications or existing health conditions. Some essential oils can interact negatively with certain medications or exacerbate existing health issues. Therefore, consulting with a qualified aromatherapist or healthcare provider before using essential oils for therapeutic purposes is always advisable.

Essential oils have a rich history and can provide health benefits; however, approaching their use through professional guidance is beneficial. Having the proper guidance and understanding of the extraction methods, dilution techniques, and potential interactions will allow the incorporation of essential oils into a holistic wellness routine safely and effectively.

Safety Precautions and Guidelines for Essential Oils

It is important to always keep essential oils safely out of reach of children and pets. Plant extracts have several beneficial uses in aromatherapy and natural healing, but they can also pose a significant danger if ingested. Essential oils come from natural sources, are highly concentrated, and should be taken with guidance. Accidental ingestion can cause serious harm to both humans and animals if improperly taken, as essential oils can be toxic and irritate the digestive system. Additionally, pets, especially cats, are more susceptible to the effects of essential oils due to their unique metabolism. Therefore, it is crucial to store essential oils securely to prevent accidental access and to educate ourselves and others about the potential risks associated with essential oils to ensure their safe and responsible use. By taking these precautions, we can enjoy the numerous benefits of essential oils while ensuring the well-being of our loved ones.

It is always important to remember to dilute essential oils before applying them topically. While they may offer many benefits, it is crucial to use caution when using them on the skin. Most essential oils should be diluted in a carrier oil such as coconut or almond oil, as applying them directly can potentially cause skin irritation or sensitivity. Carrier oils help reduce the essential oil's concentration, making it safer for use on the skin. Diluting essential oils also allows easier absorption into the skin, maximizing their therapeutic effects. When properly diluted, essential oils can promote relaxation, relieve muscle tension, improve skin health, and provide numerous other benefits. However, performing a patch test before using any new essential oil is always wise. This involves applying a small amount of diluted oil to a small skin area and monitoring for adverse reactions. By cutting essential oils and taking necessary precautions, you can enjoy their many benefits while ensuring the safety of your skin.

When introducing a new essential oil to your skincare routine, it is vital to take the necessary precautions to avoid any potential skin irritation or adverse reactions. One way to do this is by performing a patch test on a small area of your skin before applying the oil to a larger size. To do a patch test, dilute a small amount of the essential oil and use it on your inner arm. It is necessary to cut the oil to minimize the risk of any irritation or sensitization. Leave the oil on for 24 hours, carefully monitoring your skin for signs of redness, itchiness, or discomfort. This waiting period will allow you to identify potential adverse reactions and determine whether using the essential oil on a larger skin area is safe. Everyone's skin reacts differently, so it is always better to err on the side of caution and perform a patch test beforehand. By taking this simple step, you can ensure the safety and efficacy of the essential oil in your skincare routine.

When using essential oils, it is crucial to exercise caution and avoid applying them to sensitive areas such as the eyes, ears, and mucous membranes. These areas are remarkably delicate and can be easily irritated or damaged by the potent properties of essential oils. The eye area, for example, is susceptible and can be highly uncomfortable if exposed to undiluted essential oils. Similarly, the ears and mucous membranes, such as those found in the nose and mouth, can become easily irritated or inflamed if essential oils are applied directly. To ensure the safe and effective use of essential oils, it is best to dilute them properly before applying them to the skin and avoid any contact with the sensitive areas mentioned above.

When using essential oils, it is always important to prioritize your health and safety. If you have a medical condition, such as asthma, diabetes, or hypertension, it is crucial to consult with a qualified healthcare professional before incorporating essential oils into your routine. They can guide you on which oils are safe to use and whether they may interact with your medications. This is particularly important for pregnant or breastfeeding individuals, as certain essential oils can have contraindications or potential risks during these times. By seeking professional advice, you can ensure that you are using essential oils in a way that supports your overall well-being and that is compatible with any existing health considerations.

When storing essential oils, it is crucial to follow a few guidelines to ensure their longevity and effectiveness. When storing essential oils, it is best to place them in dark-colored glass bottles, protecting the oils from light exposure and degradation. Exposure to direct sunlight can break down the chemical compounds within the oils and decrease their potency. Additionally, storing essential oils in a cool and dry place is the ideal environment. This helps to prevent any moisture from entering the bottles and compromising the quality of the oils.

Therefore, moisture build-up can lead to the growth of bacteria and mold, rendering the oils ineffective or even harmful. However, keeping essential oils in a cool and dry location helps maintain the oil's potency while ensuring safety for use. Overall, by following these storage recommendations, one can prolong the shelf life of essential oils and continue to enjoy their numerous benefits for an extended period.

It is of utmost importance to exercise caution when ingesting essential oils. These potent substances should only be consumed if explicitly advised by a healthcare professional. Therefore, the reason for preventive measures is that essential oils can be toxic when ingested in significant amounts; they offer numerous health benefits when properly used. Consuming them without proper guidance can lead to adverse reactions and potential harm to the body. It is crucial to recognize that essential oils are plants' highly concentrated extracts containing potent compounds that can be harmful when not used appropriately. Therefore, internal use should only be considered under the expert supervision of a healthcare provider who can determine the appropriate dosage and suitability for your needs. Prioritizing safety and seeking professional guidance will ensure that you can enjoy the therapeutic benefits while minimizing potential risks.

When using essential oils for diffusion purposes, it is crucial to prioritize proper ventilation within the room to avoid any potential respiratory irritation. Good airflow plays a significant role in preventing any adverse effects on our respiratory system, so ensuring that windows or doors are open will allow fresh air to circulate. Additionally, it is advisable not to diffuse essential oils continuously for extended periods. While the aromatic scents of these oils can create a delightful ambiance, giving our bodies a break from the vapors to decrease prolonged exposure is essential. By practicing moderation and ensuring proper ventilation, we can enjoy the therapeutic benefits of essential oils without risking any respiratory discomfort.

When using essential oils, awareness of any potential adverse reactions that may occur is imperative. These reactions can include skin irritation, which manifests as redness, rash, or itching. If you notice any symptoms after using an essential oil, discontinue immediately. Additionally, if you experience breathing difficulties, such as shortness of breath or wheezing, it is crucial to seek medical advice as soon as possible. These symptoms could indicate an allergic reaction or respiratory irritation, which may require immediate attention. It is always better to err on the side of caution and consult a healthcare professional to ensure your safety and well-being.

When working with undiluted essential oils, it is important to exercise caution due to the potential risks associated with their handling. These oils have concentrated properties that can lead to staining surfaces, such as furniture or countertops, if accidentally spilled. Furthermore, direct contact with undiluted essential oils can irritate the skin, potentially leading to redness, itching, or even a burning sensation.

Moreover, prolonged exposure to essential oils may result in sensitization, whereby an individual's immune system becomes excessively sensitive to certain substances, resulting in adverse reactions upon further exposure. Therefore, it is crucial to take appropriate safety measures, such as wearing gloves and using proper containers, when dealing with undiluted essential oils to prevent accidents or adverse effects.

Remember, using essential oils, it is crucial to exercise caution due to their high concentration. These oils are potent and should be handled and utilized with care. Following proper safety precautions and adhering to guidelines, you can ensure the safe and effective use of essential oils, diluting them appropriately and avoiding contact with sensitive areas like the eyes and mucous membranes. Therefore, it is important to keep essential oils out of the reach of children and pets, and proper storage, such as in dark glass bottles, is also vital to preserve the oils' potency and prevent degradation. Using essential oils safely allows you to fully enjoy their numerous benefits, whether for aromatherapy, skincare, or other therapeutic purposes.

∞ ∞ ∞

Relaxation and Stress Relief Recipes

Tranquil Sleep Pillow Spray

If you're tired of tossing and turning throughout the night, desperately searching for a way to improve your sleep, look no further than a pillow spray. This incredible spray creation provides a natural, soothing solution to enhance your sleep experience. Imagine breathing in the gentle aroma of lavender or chamomile as you drift off into a peaceful slumber. This simple tranquil sleep pillow spray recipe promises to be your ticket to a more restful and rejuvenating night's sleep.

To create this magical elixir, gather a few key ingredients. Start with a base of distilled water, ensuring a pure and refreshing scent. Add a few drops of essential oil, such as lavender, renowned for its calming properties. The smell of lavender has long been associated with relaxation and tranquility, making it the perfect choice for your pillow spray. For an added touch of serenity, consider incorporating chamomile essential oil, known for its gentle and soothing effects.

Once you have collected these ingredients, combine them in a small spray bottle. Shake gently to allow the scents to blend harmoniously. Now, it's time to spritz your pillow! Just a light mist is all you need to envelop your sleep space in a cloud of tranquility. As you settle down for the night, the exquisite scent of lavender and chamomile will gently surround you, helping to calm your mind and body.

The benefits of a pillow spray extend beyond the immediate relaxation it provides. Over time, incorporating this simple ritual into your bedtime routine can signal your brain that it is time to unwind and prepare for rest. As you consistently use your sleep pillow spray, your mind will associate its scent with sleep, creating a powerful sleep-inducing trigger. The result? A more effortless and peaceful transition into dreamland.

So, try this tranquil sleep pillow spray if you're ready to bid farewell to restless nights and embrace a natural and relaxing way to enhance your sleep. You deserve the best rest possible, and with just a few simple ingredients, you can create the perfect environment for a restful and rejuvenating night's sleep. Sweet dreams await you!

Ingredients:

- 2 ounces distilled water

- 1 tablespoon witch hazel

- 10 drops of lavender essential oil

- 5 drops of chamomile essential oil

- 5 drops of cedarwood essential oil

Instructions:

1. combine the distilled water and witch hazel in a small spray bottle.

2. Add the lavender essential oil, chamomile essential oil, and cedarwood essential oil.

3. Close the spray bottle tightly and shake well to blend all the ingredients.

4. Before going to bed, spritz a few sprays of the pillow spray onto your pillow and sheets.

5. Enjoy the calming aroma as you drift off to sleep.

When using essential oils, it's important to remember that everyone has different preferences for scent strength. Therefore, feel free to adjust the quantities of essential oils used in this formula to your liking. If the recommended amount is too strong or weak for your tastes, add or reduce the number of drops accordingly. Not only can you customize the strength of the fragrance, but you can also explore other essential oils to enhance the relaxation benefits of this blend. Consider trying bergamot, ylang-ylang, or vetiver for a different aromatic experience. These oils are known for their calming properties, and incorporating them into your relaxation routine can provide a new level of tranquility and peace. So, experiment with different essential oils to find the perfect mix for your desired state of relaxation.

Calming Bath Blend

Here is a simple recipe for a calming bath blend to help you unwind and relax after a long and stressful day. The needed ingredients: one cup of Epsom salts, ten drops of lavender essential oil, and one tablespoon of coconut oil. Epsom salts are known for their ability to soothe sore muscles and relieve tension, making them the perfect base for a calming bath blend. The lavender essential oil has a calming and relaxing aroma that can help promote peace and tranquility by adding a few drops to your bath to create a soothing and aromatic experience.

Finally, the coconut oil will add a touch of moisturization to your bath, leaving your skin feeling soft and hydrated. To make this blend, combine the Epsom salts, lavender essential oil, and coconut oil until well mixed. Then, pour the mixture into a jar or container for easy use. When you're ready to take a calming bath, scoop out a handful of the blend and add it to your warm bathwater. Take a moment to breathe in the soothing scent and let all your worries melt away as you soak in the calming blend. This calming bath blend is a simple and easy way to create a spa-like experience in the comfort of your home and is the perfect addition to your self-care routine.

Ingredients:

- 1 cup Epsom salt

- 1/2 cup baking soda

- 10 drops of lavender essential oil

- 5 drops of chamomile essential oil

Instructions:

1. In a bowl, combine the Epsom salt and baking soda. Mix well to ensure they are evenly combined.

2. Add the lavender essential oil and chamomile essential oil to the bowl. Stir again to distribute the oils throughout the mixture.

3. Transfer the bath blend to a clean, airtight container for storage.

4. Add about 1/2 cup of the bath blend to a warm bath and soak for at least 20 minutes.

5. Enjoy the calming and soothing effects of lavender and chamomile in the bath when relaxing.

It is essential to take extra precautions when maintaining your skin's health and well-being. If you have sensitive skin or known allergies, it is always advisable to conduct a patch test before incorporating any new bath products into your routine. This step ensures you can identify potential adverse reactions or irritations before exposing your entire body to the product. A patch test involves applying a small amount of the product to a small area of your skin, such as the inside of your wrist or behind your ear, and monitoring it for 24 to 48 hours. By doing so, you can assess whether the product suits your skin type. This simple yet essential precaution can prevent discomfort, redness, itching, or even more severe skin conditions. Ultimately, by prioritizing your skin's unique needs, you can enjoy a more personalized bath experience while maintaining the health and vitality of your skin.

Peaceful Mind Inhaler

The Peaceful Mind Inhaler is a remarkable invention catering to individuals seeking tranquility and relief from a hectic lifestyle. Functioning as a portable aromatherapy device, this innovative creation aims to promote relaxation while effectively reducing stress. This magnificent inhaler utilizes a carefully selected blend of essential oils renowned for their calming properties, such as timeless lavender, soothing chamomile, and refreshing bergamot. Lavender's gentle aroma has been trusted for centuries for its ability to induce sleep and tranquility. Chamomile, renowned for its relaxing properties, has been used for generations to alleviate restlessness and soothe the mind. Bergamot essential oil brings a fresh and uplifting scent that helps ease tension and anxiety, providing peace and serenity. With its compact design and easy-to-use functionality, this incredible inhaler allows for on-the-go relaxation whenever and wherever one may desire. Simply inhaling the delicate blend of essential oils instantly transports users to a calm state, aiding stress and revitalizing the mind. Whether during a fragmented workday or for a dose of tranquility before sleep, the Peaceful Mind Inhaler ensures the continuous presence of inner peace, enabling individuals to navigate life's challenges with clarity and serenity.

The Peaceful Mind Inhaler is a convenient and effective way to find peace and tranquility amid a busy day. With (easy to use) design, remove the cap and bring the device close to your nostrils. As you take a deep breath through your nose, the calming aroma of the essential oils fills your senses, instantly soothing your mind. The carefully selected blend of essential oils creates a serene and relaxing atmosphere, giving you a moment of respite from the chaos of daily life. Whether you're feeling overwhelmed, stressed, or need a mental break, the Peaceful Mind Inhaler can help you find a sense of calm and tranquility. So, pause to inhale the soothing scent, and let your mind embrace the peace it deserves.

The Peaceful Mind Inhaler is designed to provide

tranquility and serenity to you on the go. Its compact size ensures that you always have it within reach, no matter where you are. Whether you carry it in your pocket, purse, or backpack, this inhaler is lightweight and portable, making it a perfect companion for daily adventures. Whenever life gets overwhelming, and stress takes its toll, reach for the Peaceful Mind Inhaler and inhale deeply; it will instantly transport you to calmness and relaxation, helping you find balance amidst the chaos. From a hectic workday to a restless night, this little inhaler grants your needed escape. And not just limited to these situations, it also proves beneficial during introspection and self-care like meditation or yoga practice. Embrace the tranquility at any time with the Peaceful Mind Inhaler, and let it guide you towards a peaceful state of mind.

The Peaceful Mind Inhaler is a remarkable product that offers numerous advantages to improving our mental well-being; by simply inhaling the calming essential oils it contains, individuals can experience a wide range of benefits. One significant advantage is its ability to reduce anxiety levels prevalent in today's fast-paced and stressful world. The soothing scents emitted by the inhaler have a powerful effect on our nervous system, helping to calm our racing thoughts and provide a sense of tranquility.

In today's fast-paced world, a good night's sleep has become a luxury for many. With our hectic schedules and endless responsibilities, it's no wonder that sleep disorders such as insomnia have become increasingly common. The Peaceful Mind Inhaler offers a much-needed solution to this issue. Its unique blend of calming scents and soothing aromas promotes relaxation and tranquility, effectively inducing a serenity conducive to deep slumber. By inhaling the therapeutic vapors, individuals struggling with sleep can finally find the respite their minds and bodies desperately crave. Imagine letting go of the day's stresses and worries, effortlessly drifting off into a world of peaceful dreams. Not only does the Peaceful Mind Inhaler help in improving sleep quality, but it also addresses the underlying factors that disrupt sleep, such as stress and an overactive mind. Its powerful formula helps to calm the mind and relax the body, allowing for a more effortless transition into a restful state.

The benefits of a good night's sleep go far beyond feeling refreshed in the morning. Adequate sleep is crucial for maintaining optimal physical and mental health; during deep sleep, the body repairs and rejuvenates, strengthens the immune system, regulates hormone levels, and supports overall well-being. By using this Peaceful Mind Inhaler, individuals can finally break free from the vicious cycle of poor sleep and exhaustion. No longer will they have to rely on sleeping pills or other pharmaceutical solutions that may come with unwanted side effects. Instead, they can turn to a natural and effective remedy that promotes healthy sleep patterns and restores balance to their life. In a world that often feels overwhelming and chaotic, the Peaceful Mind Inhaler offers a much-needed oasis of tranquility, allowing individuals to drift off into a deep and restful sleep, ready to face the challenges of a new day with renewed energy and vigor. So why continue to suffer from sleepless nights and constant fatigue when a simple solution is within reach? Try the Peaceful Mind Inhaler today and experience the transformative power of a good night's sleep.

Headaches are a common ailment that range from mild discomfort to intense pain, and they can disrupt an individual's quality of life. These headaches may arise due to various factors such as tension, sinus problems, or even stress. Regardless of the cause, the impact on one's daily routine can be considerable. This inhaler, when used, has shown promising results in alleviating headaches; however, its effectiveness is attributed to the calming properties of essential oils, which have been widely recognized for their soothing effects. By inhaling the fragrant aromas, individuals can experience quick relief and a reduction in the intense pressure often associated with headaches. This relief enables them to return to their usual activities with a clear and more focused mind. The convenience and portability of the inhaler make it an easy and practical solution for managing and minimizing the debilitating effects of headaches. Whether it is a need for instant relief or a desire to avoid relying on medication, using the inhaler can bring about quick and effective comfort, allowing individuals to regain control over their lives and the ability to function optimally.

In today's fast-paced society, finding ways to relax and relieve stress has become essential; with our hectic schedules and constant demands, it's easy to feel overwhelmed and anxious. Incorporating relaxation techniques into our daily routines is crucial for our overall well-being. And that's where the Peaceful Mind Inhaler comes in. This incredible tool offers a natural and effective way to find moments of tranquility amidst the chaos of everyday life.

The secret behind the Peaceful Mind Inhaler lies in its pure blend of calming essential oils. These oils have been carefully selected for their soothing properties, creating a blissful aroma that instantly transports you to a place of calmness and peace.

With just a few inhalations, you can feel your stress melt away with a sense of relaxation wash over you.

One of the best things about the Peaceful Mind Inhaler is its convenience; therefore, it is small and portable, making it perfect for use at work, home, or on the go. Whether you're feeling overwhelmed during a busy day at the office or need a moment to yourself in the comfort of your own home, this inhaler is always there to offer a helping hand.

But it's not just about finding temporary relief from stress. The Peaceful Mind Inhaler is a trusted companion for promoting well-being and peace in our busy lives. By incorporating the use of this inhaler into your daily routine, you can cultivate a practice of mindfulness and self-care. However, if you take a moment to breathe and focus throughout the day, it will have a profound impact on your overall mental and emotional health.

The Peaceful Mind Inhaler is a valuable tool that allows us to incorporate natural relaxation techniques into our daily lives. It provides a convenient and accessible way to find moments of tranquility no matter where we are. With its high-octane blend of calming essential oils, this inhaler is a trusted companion for promoting well-being and peace in our busy lives. So why not give yourself the gift of relaxation and serenity with the Peaceful Mind Inhaler?

It is important to be aware that while essential oils can offer numerous benefits, they can also potentially trigger allergic reactions or sensitivity in some individuals. To ensure safety, it is highly recommended to conduct a patch test before utilizing the Peaceful Mind Inhaler or any other aromatherapy product; this precautionary step allows individuals to test a small amount of the essential oil on a small area of their skin, typically the inner arm, to check for any adverse reactions before applying it more broadly.

In addition, pregnant or nursing women must exercise extra caution when using aromatherapy products. The effects of essential oils are potent, and there is a possibility that certain oils may have an impact on the health and well-being of the mother and baby; therefore, pregnant or breastfeeding mothers must consult with a healthcare professional before incorporating any aromatherapy products into their routine.

Furthermore, individuals with specific medical conditions should also seek advice from a healthcare professional before using essential oils. Some medical conditions can interact with certain oils, causing unwanted side effects or compromising existing treatments. Consulting a healthcare professional, individuals can gain valuable insights and guidance on which oils to avoid or use with caution, ensuring their well-being and minimizing potential risks.

While essential oils can offer benefits, it is crucial to exercise caution and consider the unique circumstances before incorporating them into your routine. Prioritize safety by conducting a patch test, consulting with a healthcare professional, and being aware of any personal medical conditions or pregnancy/nursing status. By doing so, individuals can enjoy the remarkable benefits of aromatherapy while minimizing the risk of adverse reactions or complications.

In today's fast-paced world, finding moments of relaxation and tranquility has become increasingly difficult. However, the Peaceful Mind Inhaler presents a brilliant solution. This small and compact inhaler is designed to promote ultimate relaxation and offer a peaceful escape from the constant chaos of our busy lives.

One of the main advantages of the Peaceful Mind Inhaler is its convenience. Its compact size makes it easy to carry in your pocket or purse, allowing access to relaxation wherever you go. Whether you're on a long commute, stuck in traffic, or need a break from the overwhelming demands of work and daily responsibilities, this inhaler can quickly transport you to tranquility.

But convenience is one of many benefits of this product. The Peaceful Mind Inhaler is also highly effective in promoting relaxation. The inhaler is infused with a carefully curated blend of essential oils proven to calm the mind and soothe the senses.

With just a few inhalations, the calming aroma of lavender, chamomile, and other relaxing scents envelopes you, melting away stress and tension.

Moreover, the Peaceful Mind Inhaler is not limited to one-time use; this inhaler is designed to last for a considerable period, ensuring moments of peace and relaxation whenever needed. This feature makes it a cost-effective and sustainable option for those seeking a reliable and convenient solution for finding serenity amidst the chaos.

Recipe for Peaceful Mind Inhaler:

Ingredients:

- 5 drops of Lavender essential oil

- 3 drops of Bergamot essential oil

- 2 drops Frankincense essential oil

- Cotton wick inhaler

Instructions:

1. Prepare a clean and dry cotton wick inhaler.

2. Carefully add five drops of Lavender essential oil to the cotton wick.

3. Add three drops of Bergamot essential oil to the same cotton wick.

4. Lastly, incorporate two drops of Frankincense essential oil onto the cotton wick.

5. Tightly close the inhaler to ensure the scent concentration is sealed.

6. To use, remove the cap, place the inhaler near your nose, and take slow, deep breaths.

The Peaceful Mind Inhaler recipe is blended perfectly with natural essential oils to create peace, serenity, and tranquility. Lavender, known for its soothing properties, gently calms the mind and helps alleviate stress and anxiety. Uplifting Bergamot adds a touch of brightness to the blend, promoting feelings of joy and revitalization. The grounding scent of Frankincense helps anchor the mind and provide a sense of stability, allowing you to find peace amidst the chaos of everyday life. This inhaler is effective but convenient; its portable design allows you to carry it wherever you go, providing instant access to its calming benefits whenever you feel overwhelmed or need a break. With just a few inhalations, you can escape from the hustle and bustle of the outside world and enter a state of relaxation and calmness. Whether at home, work, or on the go, this aroma therapy tool is always there to offer moments of tranquility and respite. Incorporate this inhaler into your daily routine and experience the power of aromatherapy in bringing peace into your life. Let the soothing aroma envelop your senses and transport you to inner stillness and harmony. With the Peaceful Mind Inhaler, serenity is just a breath away.

To continue enjoying the fragrance experience from your scented candle, it is recommended to replace the wick every few weeks when you notice a decrease in scent potency. Over time, the wick can get clogged with wax and decrease its effectiveness when releasing the fragrance into the air; therefore, by replacing the wick regularly, you will ensure that the candle burns evenly and emits a consistent scent. This simple maintenance step will guarantee that every time you light your favorite scented candle, you are greeted with a powerful and delightful aroma that fills the room. So, replacing the candle wicks regularly will make a difference in the ambiance and enjoyment provided. So be attentive to the condition of your wick, and whenever you start to notice a decline in the scent potency, be sure to swap it out for a new one. Your senses will thank you!

In conclusion, the Peaceful Mind Inhaler is a game-changer for individuals searching for moments of tranquility in their hectic lives. Its compact size, effectiveness, and long-lasting nature make it a must-have for those seeking a peaceful escape from the pressures of the modern world. With this inhaler in hand, relaxation and peace become accessible wherever you are, providing a much-needed respite from the demands of daily life.

∞ ∞ ∞

Energy and Focus Boost Recipes

Energizing Diffuser Blend

If you're looking for an energizing aroma to invigorate your senses and boost your productivity, look no further than this delightful diffuser blend recipe. Combining essential oils known for their uplifting properties, this blend creates an atmosphere of vitality and freshness in any room. This rejuvenating blend is created by combining a few drops of peppermint, lemon, and rosemary essential oils into your diffuser.

The peppermint's crisp and cooling scent will awaken your mind and increase focus, while the bright and citrusy notes of lemon will promote feelings of clarity and alertness. The rosemary's woody and herbaceous aroma will provide mental clarity and enhance cognitive performance. Together, these oils work harmoniously to create a powerful blend that will leave you feeling revitalized and ready to tackle any task that comes your way; so, give this energizing diffuser blend a try and experience the uplifting benefit for yourself.

- 3 drops of Peppermint essential oil: Peppermint is known for its uplifting properties, promoting mental clarity and energy.

- 3 drops of Lemon essential oil: Lemon has a bright and refreshing scent that can help to invigorate and energize the mind and body.

- 2 drops of Rosemary essential oil: Rosemary is a stimulating and revitalizing oil known for improving focus and clarity.

- 2 drops of Sweet Orange essential oil: Sweet Orange has a

naturally uplifting and mood-boosting scent, making it a great addition to an energizing blend.

If you want to enhance your living or workspace with a refreshing and energizing atmosphere, try using a diffuser. Combine a few essential oils with water to create a refreshing aroma that will elevate the mood and energy levels within your surroundings. If you want to boost productivity in your home office, create a welcoming ambiance in your living room, and the possibilities are endless. With their natural aromatherapy properties, essential oils have been used for centuries to promote relaxation, uplift spirits, and improve overall well-being. So, why not bring this ancient practice into your life and experience the benefits firsthand? By simply adding a few drops of your favorite essential oils, such as citrusy lemon, refreshing peppermint, or uplifting eucalyptus, to a diffuser filled with water, you can fill your space with an aromatic symphony that will awaken your senses and inspire productivity. So go ahead, let the refreshing and energizing scents envelop your space and transform it into a haven of positive energy and tranquility.

Here is a recipe for an energizing diffuser blend:

Ingredients:

- 3 drops of peppermint essential oil

- 3 drops of rosemary essential oil

- 2 drops of lemon essential oil

Instructions:

1. Fill your diffuser with water according to the manufacturer's instructions.

2. Add the specified number of drops of each essential oil to the water in the diffuser.

3. Turn on the diffuser and enjoy the refreshing scent that fills your space.

Note: Essential oils are highly concentrated and should be used with caution. Follow any safety guidelines and consult a professional with any concerns or questions.

Refreshing Citrus Body Scrub

Ingredients:

- 1 cup of sugar

- ¼ cup of coconut oil (melted)

- Zest from 1 lemon

- Zest from 1 orange

- 10-12 drops of lemon essential oil

- 10-12 drops of orange essential oil

Instructions:

1. combine the sugar and melted coconut oil in a medium-sized bowl. Mix well to form a paste-like consistency.

2. Add the lemon and orange zest to the bowl and stir until well combined.

3. Slowly add the drops of lemon and orange essential oil, stirring continuously.

4. Transfer the mixture to an airtight container and store it in

a cool, dry place.

5. To use, scoop out a small amount of the scrub and gently massage it onto damp skin in circular motions. Rinse thoroughly with warm water.

6. Enjoy the refreshing citrus scent and the smooth, exfoliated skin!

This recipe offers the unique opportunity to customize your ideal scrub to match your preferences. Whether you desire a coarser or finer scrub, the sugar used in the recipe can be easily adjusted. Add more sugar to the mixture if you crave a more invigorating exfoliation experience. This will provide a heightened scrubbing sensation, perfect for individuals who enjoy a more intense exfoliation.

Alternatively, if you prefer a gentler scrub, you can decrease the amount of sugar or even grind it into a finer texture. This alteration will result in a milder exfoliation, particularly beneficial for sensitive skin or seeking a more subtle scrubbing effect. The true beauty of this recipe lies within its adaptability, granting you the power to create a scrub that flawlessly suits your unique skin care needs and preferences.

Mental Clarity Rollerball Blend

The Mental Clarity Rollerball Blend is expertly crafted using a precise combination of essential oils chosen to enhance mental focus, concentration, and clarity. This remarkable blend is a carefully curated selection of ingredients that promote a clear and focused mind.

The first ingredient in this incredible blend is rosemary essential oil. Known for its stimulating properties, rosemary has long been recognized for its enhanced memory and cognitive function. Its refreshing scent helps to awaken the senses, promoting alertness and mental clarity. Another essential oil in this remarkable blend is peppermint. With its refreshing and cooling aroma, peppermint essential oil helps to stimulate mental alertness and increase concentration. It is also known to aid in relieving mental fatigue, allowing for improved mental clarity and focus.

Lemon essential oil is another ingredient in this blend. Thanks to its uplifting and energizing properties, lemon essential oil enhances mental clarity and improves mood. Its fresh and citrusy scent helps to create a sense of clarity and focus, making it an excellent choice for mental well-being.

Next, the Mental Clarity Rollerball Blend includes basil essential oil. With its warm and herbaceous aroma, basil essential oil has been used for centuries for its ability to promote mental focus and improve concentration. It is also known for its relaxing properties, helping to reduce stress and mental tension.

Finally, the blend is bound with a carrier oil, such as jojoba or fractionated coconut oil, to dilute the essential oils and make it safe for topical application. This allows for easy and convenient use of the Mental Clarity Rollerball Blend, ensuring remarkable benefits can be enjoyed anytime, anywhere.

In conclusion, the Mental Clarity Rollerball Blend is an

extraordinary combination of essential oils designed to enhance mental focus, concentration, and clarity. With its meticulous selection of ingredients, this blend promotes a clear and focused mind, helping you to tackle tasks with precision and efficiency. Embracing these essential oils using the Mental Clarity Rollerball Blend and experience the incredible benefits.

- 10 drops of Rosemary essential oil: Known for enhancement of memory and cognitive function, rosemary essential oil is an ingredient in this blend.

- 10 drops of Peppermint essential oil: Peppermint is stimulating and invigorating, helping to increase alertness and mental clarity.

- 5 drops of Lemon essential oil: Lemon oil is refreshing and uplifting, providing an energetic boost to the mind.

- 5 drops of Frankincense essential oil: Frankincense is grounding and calming, helping to reduce mental distractions and improve focus.

- A carrier oil (such as fractionated coconut oil) to dilute the essential oils and make them safe for direct application.

Creating your essential oil blend is a fun and easy way to personalize your aromatherapy experience. All you need is a 10ml rollerball bottle, some essential oils (of your choice), and carrier oil. Start by carefully adding the specified number of drops for each essential oil into the rollerball bottle. The number of essential oil drops (will depend on the specific blend you are creating) required for the recipe or guideline. Once the essential oils are added, fill the rest of the bottle with your chosen carrier oil. Leave a small space at the top to ensure room for the rollerball top to be inserted. Once the rollerball is in place, securely screw on the cap. Now, it's time to give your blend a good shake. Gently mix the oils by shaking the bottle back and forth. This will ensure that the essential oils and carrier oil are thoroughly combined. Once your blend is mixed, it's ready to use. Apply the rollerball directly to your skin to enjoy the benefits of your custom essential oil blend.

The rollerball blend is a convenient and effective way to boost mental clarity and focus. Apply a few drops to your temples, wrists, or behind your ears, and you'll experience instant invigoration. The powerful aroma of the blend will envelop your senses, awakening your mind and helping you feel more alert. As you take a deep breath, you'll feel the refreshing scent working its magic, clearing any mental fog and enhancing your cognitive abilities. Whether you're studying for an important exam, tackling a challenging project at work, or need a mental pick-me-up during the day, this rollerball blend is your go-to solution. Its quick and easy application makes it ideal for on-the-go use, so you can always have it by your side to access its powerful benefits whenever needed. So go ahead and indulge in the aromatic goodness of this rollerball blend and experience the mental boost and enhanced focus it brings to your life.

When it comes to essential oils, it is vital to remember that they are highly concentrated and, therefore, require careful usage. This calls for a cautious approach to ensure their safe and practical application. It is essential to exercise caution if you are pregnant, nursing, or if you have any preexisting medical conditions. In such instances, it is strongly advised to consult with a healthcare professional before incorporating any essential oil blend into your routine. This step can help address any concerns or risks associated with your unique circumstances, ensuring the safest possible experience. By seeking guidance from a healthcare professional, you can confidently navigate the world of essential oils and make informed decisions about their usage based on your needs and health considerations.

Here is a recipe for a mental clarity rollerball blend:

Ingredients:

- 10 drops of peppermint essential oil

- 10 drops of rosemary essential oil

- 5 drops of lemon essential oil

- 5 drops of frankincense essential oil

- Carrier oil (such as fractionated coconut oil or jojoba oil)

Instructions:

1. add peppermint, rosemary, lemon, and frankincense essential oils in a small glass rollerball bottle.

2. Fill the rest of the bottle with your chosen carrier oil.

3. Secure the rollerball top onto the bottle and gently shake to mix the oils.

4. To use, apply the blend to your temples, wrists, or back of your neck whenever you need mental clarity.

Essential oils are potent substances that require careful handling and consideration. Due to their high concentration, it is crucial to exercise caution when using them. Before applying essential oils to the skin, it is necessary to be aware of any allergies or sensitivities. To ensure safety, conducting a patch test before applying the oil blend to larger areas of the body is recommended. This process involves using a small amount of the oil on a small skin patch and monitoring for any adverse reactions, such as redness, itching, or swelling. By performing a patch test, individuals can identify potential sensitivities and avoid skin irritations or problems. This precautionary step provides peace of mind and allows one to enjoy the benefits of essential oils without any unnecessary risks.

∞ ∞ ∞

Mood Uplifting Recipes

Joyful Room Spray

J oyful Room Spray is a remarkable product that brings joy and happiness to every room. Its blend of invigorating and revitalizing scents is formulated to uplift your mood and create a positive and harmonious atmosphere throughout the space. With every spritz of Joyful Room Spray, you can instantly experience a burst of refreshing fragrances that awaken your senses, lifting your spirits and brightening your day. This extraordinary room spray transforms any ordinary space into a sanctuary of bliss and contentment, where stress and worries are effortlessly replaced with an overwhelming sense of joy and tranquility. From the delicate and enchanting floral notes that transport you to a serene garden to the zesty citrus-infused essences that invigorate your senses, Joyful Room Spray encompasses scents that cater to different preferences and occasions. Whether you are preparing for a social gathering, looking to create a peaceful ambiance for relaxation, or simply wanting to infuse your living space with a touch of happiness, this exceptional product is designed to cater to all your needs. So, indulge in the enchanting aroma of Joyful Room Spray, and let it fill your surroundings with happiness and positivity.

The room spray is crafted with utmost attention to detail using the best ingredients. Each component has been carefully chosen for its ability to enhance the overall ambiance of any space. With this room spray, you can transform your home or office into a haven of tranquility and freshness. The delightful fragrance combination of citrusy, floral, and woody notes is perfect. The blend is expertly formulated to ensure the spray emits a harmonious and joyful aroma that instantly uplifts your mood.

Citrusy tones add energy and vibrancy, while floral undertones provide a soothing atmosphere. The woody notes help to ground the fragrance, creating a sense of stability and warmth. This room spray is a must-have for anyone who wants to create a welcoming and rejuvenating environment. Whether it is to refresh your living room, bedroom, or workspace, this spray elevates the ambiance to new heights. Experience the magic of this exceptional room spray, and let its refreshing scent envelop your surroundings in a luxurious embrace.

Fragrances such as orange or lemon (called citrusy notes) can have a refreshing impact, which awakens the senses and provides an instant burst of energy. Think of the zesty scent of freshly squeezed oranges or the tangy aroma of lemons - they instantly uplift the mood and feel revitalized.

On the other end of the fragrance spectrum, we have the

floral notes, which infuse delicate fragrances like jasmine or rose to exude elegance and softness. These elegant fragrances create an atmosphere where jasmine transports you to an enchanting garden while the aroma of roses evokes love and tenderness.

Lastly, let's remember the woody notes. The fragrances of cedarwood or sandalwood provide a sense of grounding and warmth. These scents have a way of creating a cozy and comforting ambiance. Imagine the earthy and rich aroma of cedarwood that brings to mind a walk through a peaceful forest or the creamy and creamy undertones of sandalwood that envelop you in a soothing embrace.

Together, these three categories of fragrances create a harmonious blend that can transport you to different moods and environments. Whether you need an energizing boost, looking for elegance, or seeking a sense of grounding, the combination of citrusy, floral, and woody notes can cater to your every desire.

Using Joyful Room Spray is a breeze, as it requires minimal

effort. All you have to do is give the bottle a few spritzes in the air or on fabrics, and voila! The delightful and refreshing scent will effortlessly permeate the entire room. This versatile spray can be used in any home, making it easy to infuse a cheerful ambiance wherever you go. It's not limited to just the confines of your living space either; bring Joyful Room Spray to your office and let it elevate the mood of your workspace, or even keep it in your car to create a positive and inviting environment during your daily commute. The options are endless with this refreshing and uplifting spray, making it a must-have addition to your everyday life.

Joyful Room Spray is a truly versatile product that caters to every need. Its vibrant and uplifting fragrance is particularly beneficial in the morning when we often need an extra boost to kick-start our day. By spraying it around your living space, you can instantly create a revitalizing atmosphere that invigorates your senses and revives your energy. Delightful room spray enhances your mood as the day passes, keeping you motivated and positive, even during the most demanding tasks. Its carefully selected blend of scents has the power to uplift and promote relaxation, allowing you to find a sense of calm amidst the chaos of daily life. Whether it's a busy workday or a lazy weekend, Joyful Room Spray can transform your environment into a sanctuary of tranquility, leaving you feeling refreshed and rejuvenated. Therefore, this delightful spray is not limited to personal use; it also serves as a tool for creating a joyful ambiance for special occasions. Whether hosting a party, welcoming guests, or celebrating a milestone, a few spritzes of Joyful Room Spray can instantly uplift the mood and set the tone for a memorable and delightful experience. It adds a touch of joy and positivity to any gathering, making everyone feel relaxed, happy, and ready to celebrate. With Joyful Room Spray as your companion, you can always count on an instant pick-me-up, no matter the time or the occasion.

Recipe for a Joyful Room Spray:

Ingredients:

- 2 ounces of distilled water

- 1 tablespoon of vodka or witch hazel

- 10 drops of sweet orange essential oil

- 10 drops of lemon essential oil

- 5 drops of bergamot essential oil

Instructions:

1. combine the distilled water and vodka/witch hazel in a small spray bottle.

2. Add the sweet orange, lemon, and bergamot essential oils to the mixture.

3. Securely close the spray bottle and shake well to blend all ingredients thoroughly.

4. give the bottle another gentle shake before using it to ensure everything is evenly distributed.

5. Spray this uplifting room spray into any area of your home

that could use a fresh and joyful scent.

It is important to note that this product contains natural ingredients, which may tend to separate over time. Therefore, it is recommended to shake the product well before each use. This step is crucial to ensure that all the ingredients are evenly distributed and that the product functions effectively. By shaking the product, any possible separation that may have occurred is addressed, and the formulation is restored to its optimal state. This preventive measure guarantees that the product delivers its intended benefits and maintains its high quality. Shaking the product well before each use is a simple yet necessary step to ensure the user's best possible experience and results.

Enjoy the refreshing aroma of this homemade Joyful Room Spray!

Happy Roller Blend

The Happy Roller Blend is a remarkable blend of essential oils carefully selected to enhance feelings of happiness, joy, and positivity. This incredible blend has been created by combining a harmonious combination of various oils renowned for their uplifting properties. This blend's aromatic essence can instantly uplift the mood, promoting inner peace and contentment.

The Happy Roller Blend consists of a perfect combination of essential oils, each contributing its unique properties to the overall blend. With sweet and citrusy notes, the mix includes oils such as uplifting bergamot, refreshing grapefruit, and revitalizing lemon. These oils are well-known for their ability to promote a sense of positivity and boost one's overall well-being.

Additionally, the blend incorporates the soothing scent of lavender, which is renowned for its calming effects on the mind and body. Combined with the joyful aroma of orange, the Happy Roller Blend creates a refreshing and calming experience, allowing one to embrace a more positive mindset.

The blend can be easily created by combining these oils in precise quantities, offering a delightful sensory experience. Once crafted, it can be applied to the pulse points or used in a diffuser to fill the space with its refreshing aroma. Whether used as a personal fragrance or for creating a serene atmosphere, the Happy Roller Blend is the perfect companion for those seeking to infuse their lives with happiness and joy. Experience the transformative power of this remarkable blend and invite a wave of positivity into your daily life.

- 10 drops of Bergamot essential oil: Bergamot has a citrusy and uplifting aroma that is often used to boost mood and reduce feelings of stress and anxiety.

- 8 drops of Lemon essential oil: Lemon oil has a fresh and energizing scent that can help uplift and enhance mood. It is also known for its cleansing and purifying properties.

- 6 drops of Ylang Ylang essential oil: Ylang Ylang has a sweet, floral aroma that is often used to promote a sense of relaxation, happiness, and joy. It is also known to help reduce stress and anxiety.

- 4 drops of Grapefruit essential oil: Grapefruit oil has a refreshing and citrusy scent that can help lift mood and promote a positive outlook. It is also known for its energizing and uplifting properties.

- 2 drops of Frankincense essential oil: Frankincense has a woody and earthy aroma that promotes calmness, relaxation, and spiritual well-being.

To create the uplifting and mood-boosting Happy Roller Blend, you can effortlessly gather the specified essential oils and blend them in a roller bottle. These carefully selected essential oils have been thoughtfully combined to create a harmonious aroma that promotes happiness and positivity. To complete the blend, fill the roller bottle with carrier oil (such as fractionated coconut or sweet almond oil), which will help to distribute the essential oils onto your skin.

Once you have successfully prepared the Happy Roller Blend, you have a convenient and portable mood-enhancing companion at your fingertips. Whether you're facing a challenging day at work or need an emotional pick-me-up, this delightful blend can be easily rolled onto your wrists, temples, or behind your ears. Before applying, inhale the soothing and refreshing fragrance, allowing it to envelop your senses and uplift your spirits. The carefully selected oils work synergistically to awaken joy, positivity, and happiness within you.

By incorporating the Happy Roller Blend into your daily routine, you can effortlessly infuse your day with happiness and enthusiasm. The mood-boosting properties of this blend can provide an antidote to stress, anxiety, or low mood as a gentle reminder to prioritize your emotional well-being. Embrace the benefits of these essential oils, allowing their natural properties to enhance your mood and provide you with a renewed sense of contentment and joy. So, enjoy the uplifting and exhilarating

Note: Essential oils are highly concentrated and should be used with caution. It is recommended that you do a patch test before you apply any new blends to your skin. If irritation occurs, discontinue use. Women pregnant, nursing, or those with health concerns, please consult with healthcare professionals before using essential oils.

Blissful Bath Soak

Blissful Bath Soak – it's a lavish indulgence that transports you to a serene oasis of tranquility within the comfort of your bathroom. Crafted with the utmost care and attention to detail, this luxurious creation of only the finest natural ingredients. The soothing essential oils, carefully selected botanical extracts, and therapeutic Epsom salts work harmoniously to create a truly blissful and immersive bathing experience.

The potent combination of these ingredients is designed

to provide remarkable respite for your body and mind. As you enter the warm water, your stress and worries melt away; the gentle scent of the essential oil envelopes you in a cocoon of serenity, allowing you to embrace a moment of relaxation.

But Blissful Bath Soak is not limited to mere relaxation. Its powerful formula goes beyond simply providing a temporary escape. The Epsom salts work wonders in easing muscle tension and soreness, providing much-needed relief after a long day or an intense workout. Meanwhile, the carefully chosen botanical extracts nourish and rejuvenate your skin, leaving it soft, supple, and gloriously pampered.

Blissful Bath Soak can promote a sense of calm and wellness, enriching divine creation, mind-clearing, and worries fade into the background. A sense of peacefulness washes over you, restoring balance to your inner self. The restorative powers of Blissful Bath Soak are underestimated – it can rejuvenate your body and spirit.

Indulge in the luxury of Blissful Bath Soak and discover a

whole new level of blissful bathing. Let go of the outside world and allow yourself the luxury of pure relaxation. Embrace the transformative power of this magnificent creation, and emerge from your bath feeling rejuvenated, refreshed, and ready to face the world with a newfound sense of calm and tranquility.

To experience the full benefits of Blissful Bath Soak, it is recommended to follow a few simple steps. Begin by filling your bathtub with warm water, ensuring your temperature preference. Once the tub is filled, take a moment to take in the delightful scent of the bath soak, allowing yourself to feel excited about the relaxation that awaits. With a generous hand, add the desired amount of Blissful Bath Soak into the running water as it dissolves into a fragrant, colorful swirl. As the soothing aroma fills the air, take a deep breath and step into the tub, allowing the water to envelop your body. The moment you immerse yourself in the bath, you will feel a sense of tranquility and calm wash over you. With your eyes closed, let the therapeutic properties of carefully selected ingredients work on your skin and senses. As you settle into the warm embrace of the bath, take this time to escape from the stresses of daily life and truly unwind. Feel the tension melt away from your muscles as the gentle heat of the water penetrates your body, leaving you feeling refreshed and revived. Allow yourself to luxuriate in the experience, allowing your mind to relax and recharge. So, after a long day or a regular self-care ritual, Blissful Bath Soak provides a moment of pure bliss and rejuvenating benefits that this bath soak offers.

Blissful Bath Soak is a luxury bath with Epsom salts for tired muscles and joints. Epsom salts have long been known for their ability to relax and soothe aching bodies. As you soak in the warm water, the salts work their magic, relieving tension and allowing for a deep sense of relaxation to take over.

But the benefits continue beyond there. The essential oils infused in this bath soak provide aromatherapy benefits, elevating the entire bath experience. The soothing scents can envelop your senses, creating a serene atmosphere that uplifts your mood and washes away the day's stress. When choosing a lavender-infused blend for a calming effect or a citrus scent to invigorate your senses, these essential oils enhance the relaxation and rejuvenation of your bath.

In addition to the Epsom salts and essential oils, Blissful Bath Soak contains botanical extracts that nourish and soften your skin. As you immerse yourself in the warm water, these extracts work their magic, leaving your skin feeling silky smooth and deeply moisturized. Gone are the days of dry and dull skin after a bath - with Blissful Bath Soak, your skin will feel rejuvenated and radiant.

In conclusion, Blissful Bath Soak is a must-have addition to your self-care routine. With its blend of Epsom salts, essential oils, and botanical extracts, this bath soak offers a truly blissful experience that relaxes the body and mind. So go ahead, indulge in a long soak, and let the stress melt away as you emerge rejuvenated, with soft, nourished skin and a sense of calm and tranquility like never before.

This Blissful Bath Soak recipe will take your self-care routine to another level. Whether you've had a long and tiring day or want to treat yourself to some much-needed pampering, this bath soak is a must-have. Designed to transform your bathroom into a peaceful sanctuary, it allows you to escape from the chaos of everyday life and immerse yourself in pure serenity. As you pour the silky-smooth blend into your bath, the soothing aroma fills the air, immediately transporting you to tranquility. Close your eyes and feel the stress and tension slowly melt away as you sink into the warm water. The luxurious formula of the Blissful Bath Soak nourishes and hydrates your skin, leaving it feeling silky, soft, and rejuvenated. Every minute in this blissful bath feels like a lavish spa experience, and you will emerge from the tub feeling refreshed, revitalized, and completely relaxed. Treat yourself to this little slice of heaven and let the troubles of the outside world fade away as you indulge in the ultimate self-care ritual with the Blissful Bath Soak.

Blissful Bath Soak Recipe

Ingredients:

- 1 cup Epsom salt

- 1/2 cup baking soda

- 10 drops of lavender essential oil

- 5 drops of chamomile essential oil

- 3 tablespoons dried rose petals

Instructions:

1. In a bowl, combine the Epsom salt and baking soda.

2. Add the lavender essential oil and chamomile essential oil to the mixture. Stir well to ensure even distribution.

3. Gently fold in the dried rose petals.

4. Transfer the bath soak mixture to an airtight container for storage.

To use:

1. Fill your bathtub with warm water.

2. Add half a cup of the blissful bath soak mixture to the water.

3. Stir the water with your hand to help dissolve the ingredients.

4. Relax and soak in the bath for at least 20 minutes.

It is essential to prioritize your health and safety, especially regarding skincare products. That is why performing a patch test before using a bath soak is highly recommended if you have any known allergies or skin sensitivities. You can assess potential adverse reactions by applying a small amount of the product on a small area of your skin, such as your inner arm. This proactive step allows you to identify any allergic reactions or irritations that may occur, allowing you to avoid any discomfort or harm from using a full bath soak. Taking this precaution ensures you can enjoy a relaxing and nourishing bathing experience without any negative consequences, allowing you to prioritize your skin's health and well-being.

Enjoy this luxurious and soothing bath experience created just for you!

∞ ∞ ∞

Immunity Support Recipes

Germ-Fighting Hand Sanitizer

Germ-Fighting Hand Sanitizer is an essential product in our daily lives that acts as a powerful weapon against invisible enemies lurking on our hands. This efficient product is designed to swiftly eliminate, kill, or significantly decrease the number of harmful germs on our hands. Boasting a formidable composition, Germ-Fighting Hand Sanitizer primarily contains alcohol, characterized by isopropyl alcohol or ethanol. These potent ingredients have been scientifically proven to exhibit unparalleled effectiveness in exterminating a broad spectrum of bacteria and viruses that make their way onto our precious hands. Keeping this invaluable product within arm's reach ensures that we can maintain the highest hygiene, protecting ourselves and those around us from the potential threat of infectious diseases.

Hand sanitizers have become an indispensable part of our daily lives, serving as a convenient alternative to soap and water in situations where their immediate availability might be lacking. This product has gained immense popularity in healthcare facilities and public places, where the potential risk of spreading germs is heightened due to the constant influx of people. Hand sanitizers have proven to be a crucial tool in combating infectious diseases, particularly during robust flu seasons when the transmission of germs is at its peak. Through their highly effective germ-killing formula, these sanitizers act as a reliable and efficient defense mechanism against harmful bacteria and viruses. By emphasizing the importance of regular hand hygiene and the use of hand sanitizers, we can collectively contribute to preventing the spread of illnesses and maintaining a healthier and safer environment for ourselves and those around us.

With germ-fighting hand sanitizer, it is crucial to follow these steps for optimal results. First, dispense a small amount, approximately equivalent to a dime-sized drop, onto the palm of your hand. Next, vigorously rub the sanitizer onto the surfaces of both hands, ensuring to cover all areas thoroughly; however, it is necessary to pay attention to the fingertips, nails, and spaces between fingers, as these are usually ignored parts that harbor germs. The friction created during the rubbing process aids in breaking down any potential pathogens or bacteria on your hands. Continue rubbing until the sanitizer evaporates to indicate it has effectively done its job. This simple and quick process is an excellent way to maintain good hand hygiene, especially when soap and water are not readily available. Incorporating hand sanitizer into your daily routine is an outstanding preventive measure against the transmission of germs and illnesses, keeping you and those around you safe and healthy.

Hand sanitizers have gained popularity because of their effectiveness in killing various germs, which has become vital in maintaining good hygiene, especially when soap and water are not readily available. However, it is essential to note that hand sanitizers may be less effective in removing types of contaminants, such as chemicals or heavy metals. While they excel in eliminating harmful bacteria, viruses, and fungi, these sanitizers may not have the capability to get rid of other damaging substances. In such cases, it is crucial that washing hands thoroughly with soap and water not only can one physically remove dirt and germs from their hands, but it also helps to break down and wash away any chemical or heavy metal residues that pose a health risk. Therefore, it is essential to understand that although hand sanitizers are beneficial and convenient, they can only partially replace the importance of thorough handwashing with soap and water when dealing with specific varieties of contaminants.

When it comes to hand sanitizers, it is vital to remember that they are all different because some may not be as effective as others, which makes it crucial to choose the right product. The Centers for Disease Control and Prevention (CDC) advises that hand sanitizers should contain at least 60% alcohol; therefore, the CDC has recommended this concentration to maximize effectiveness in fighting germs and preventing the spread of diseases. By using hand sanitizers with the recommended alcohol content, you can feel more confident in your efforts to maintain personal hygiene and minimize the risk of getting sick. Whether it's when we're on the go or in situations where soap and water are not easily accessible, right-hand sanitizer can play a significant role in keeping us safe and healthy.

Germ-fighting hand sanitizers have become integral to our daily lives, offering an accessible and efficient solution to sustain suitable hand hygiene. With their quick-drying formulas and portable packaging, these sanitizers have gained immense popularity in reducing the transmission of germs. They are especially beneficial when soap and water are not readily available, such as during travel or while out and about in public places. However, it is crucial to remember that hand sanitizers should never be used as a substitute for regular handwashing with soap and water. While they can effectively kill many germs and bacteria, they may not effectively remove visible dirt, grease, or harmful chemicals that can linger on our hands. Therefore, it remains important to continue practicing proper handwashing techniques, especially when our hands are visibly dirty or greasy. By combining the use of hand sanitizers and regular handwashing, we can ensure thorough hand cleanliness and minimize the risk of spreading infections. So, let's embrace the convenience of hand sanitizers while prioritizing the traditional handwashing method, as both work hand-in-hand to keep us healthy and safe.

On this occasion, I would like to present a recipe for a

highly effective hand sanitizer that aids in the fight against germs.

Ingredients:

- 2/3 cup of rubbing alcohol (99% isopropyl alcohol)

- 1/3 cup of Aloe Vera gel

- Optional: Essential oils for fragrance (such as lavender or tea tree oil)

Instructions:

1. Begin by ensuring that your hands and all utensils are clean.

2. In a small bowl, combine the rubbing alcohol and Aloe Vera gel thoroughly. This mixture will serve as the base for our hand sanitizer.

3. If desired, add a few drops of essential oil for a pleasant scent. Be sure to choose oils that have antibacterial properties if you prefer an extra germ-fighting boost.

4. Stir all ingredients together until they are well blended.

5. Using a funnel, carefully transfer the sanitizer into empty bottles or containers that can be sealed tightly.

6. Apply a small amount to your hands whenever soap and water are not readily available, and rub it in thoroughly until dry.

This homemade hand sanitizer can effectively combat germs, but it should not replace regular handwashing with soap and water.

In conclusion, this recipe proves helpful in keeping you and those around you safe from harmful germs. Stay vigilant and maintain good hygiene practices!

Winter Immunity Inhaler

The Winter Immunity Inhaler is a revolutionary device specifically designed to assist individuals in strengthening their immune systems and warding off common winter ailments. Infused with a blend of essential oils and natural ingredients, this advanced inhaler acts as a protective shield against seasonal illnesses. Seamlessly resembling a regular inhaler, the Winter Immunity Inhaler deviates from conventional medication by delivering a unique blend of botanical extracts through inhalation. This advanced technology offers a straightforward method for uplifting the body's natural immunities during the winter months; however, with its effortless application and potential benefits, the Winter Immunity Inhaler is a promising solution for individuals seeking enhanced immune support to combat the challenges that the colder season brings.

When it comes to the formulation of products, such as air fresheners or cleaning solutions, the specific ingredients and blend can vary based on the brand or product. However, a common thread among these products is the inclusion of essential oils, which provide various benefits. These oils, including eucalyptus, peppermint, lavender, tea tree, and lemon, are renowned for their antiviral and antibacterial properties. By harnessing the natural power of these oils, these products aim to reduce the risk of catching a cold or flu. Eucalyptus, for instance, is commonly known for its ability to ease respiratory issues, making it a popular choice for products intended to prevent illness. Peppermint has an uplifting aroma, helps cleanse the air, and produces a cooling feeling to alleviate discomfort. Lavender is celebrated for its relaxation properties and helps create a calming environment. Tea tree oil has potent antimicrobial properties and is a natural disinfectant, thus promoting a hygienic atmosphere. Lastly, the refreshing scent of lemon adds a refreshing touch to these products but may also contribute to a cleaner and more revitalizing space. Overall, these carefully selected essential oils form the backbone of these products, providing both a delightful fragrance and potential health benefits.

In the winter season, our respiratory system gets compromised from the dry air and tends to develop congestion, which blocks our nasal passages, making it difficult to breathe. This is where the Winter Immunity Inhaler comes in. This innovative product harnesses the power of aromatic vapors to provide relief and promote easier breathing. Inhaling these soothing vapors opens our nasal passages and clears the airways for more efficient airflow. Not only does this help alleviate congestion, but it also provides an immune boost. The inhaler is specially designed to deliver these healing vapors directly to the respiratory system, where they can work their magic. It is recommended to use the inhaler a few times a day or whenever the need arises for an immune system boost. Whether you're struggling with a stubborn cold or wanting to stay healthy during the winter months, the Winter Immunity Inhaler can be a helpful ally in promoting better respiratory health and overall well-being.

When it comes to finding relief during the winter months, many individuals have found comfort in using a Winter Immunity Inhaler. However, it is crucial to acknowledge that there is still a lack of comprehensive scientific research regarding the specific effects of these products. While some people swear by the benefits they have experienced with these inhalers, it is always advisable to exercise caution and consult with a healthcare professional before incorporating any natural remedy into your routine. This is particularly important if you have pre-existing conditions or are taking other medications. By seeking medical guidance, you can ensure that the Winter Immunity Inhaler is safe and compatible with your health situation. Remember, prioritizing your well-being should always be the top priority, and professional advice can provide you with the necessary assurance and guidance in making informed decisions about your health.

Here is a recipe for a winter immunity inhaler:

Ingredients:

- 5 drops of eucalyptus essential oil

- 3 drops of tea tree essential oil

- 2 drops of peppermint essential oil

- 2 drops of lemon essential oil

Instructions:

1. Combine all the essential oils in a small glass bottle.

2. Close the lid tightly and shake well to mix the oils.

3. Take off the lid and place the inhaler tube over it.

4. Inhale deeply through each nostril, holding each breath for a few seconds before exhaling.

5. Repeat this process throughout the day to boost your immunity during winter.

Note: Essential oils can be vital, so if you have any sensitivities or allergies, please consult a healthcare professional before using this inhaler.

Defense Diffuser Blend

A defense diffuser blend is a powerful combination of essential oils specifically formulated to fortify the immune system and provide protection against a wide range of airborne germs and bacteria. This blend acts as a shield, creating a healthier environment and reducing the chances of falling ill due to respiratory infections or other diseases caused by airborne pathogens. The recipe for this defense diffuser blend entails carefully selecting essential oils known for their antiviral, antimicrobial, and immune-boosting properties.

These oils work synergistically to enhance the body's natural defense mechanisms, making it more resilient against harmful microbes and boosting overall well-being. By diffusing this blend, you can create a refreshing and germ-free atmosphere, promoting better respiratory health and supporting a robust immune system. It is vital to note that while a defense diffuser blend can have significant benefits, it should not replace other preventive measures such as proper hygiene practices or medical advice. Regularly using this blend with a healthy lifestyle can help safeguard your health and promote overall wellness.

- 3 drops of Tea Tree essential oil: It is known for its antimicrobial and antiviral properties, making it a great addition to any defense blend.

- 3 drops of Eucalyptus essential oil: Eucalyptus oil has antibacterial and antiviral properties that can help purify the air and support a healthy immune system.

- 2 drops of Lemon essential oil: Lemon oil is known for its cleansing properties and can help purify the air, making it a great addition to a defense blend.

- 2 drops of Frankincense essential oil: Frankincense oil has immune-boosting properties that can help protect against germs and bacteria.

- 1 drop of Rosemary essential oil: Rosemary oil has antimicrobial properties that can help purify the air and support a healthy immune system.

To use the defense diffuser blend, all you need to do is add the exact number of drops of each essential oil to your diffuser and follow the manufacturer's instructions. It's such a simple and convenient way to enjoy the benefits of this potent blend. Once the diffuser is set up correctly, you can enjoy the wonderful aroma filling your home or office. Not only will it make your space smell amazing, but it will also provide you with a natural defense against airborne germs. By diffusing this blend, you can boost your immunity and create a protective barrier that will help safeguard you and your loved ones from potential illnesses. It's a great addition to your self-care routine, especially when staying healthy and protected is paramount.

Recipe for Defense Diffuser Blend:

Ingredients:

- 3 drops of Tea Tree essential oil

- 2 drops of Eucalyptus essential oil

- 2 drops of Lemon essential oil

- 1 drop of Rosemary essential oil

Instructions:

1. add the required number of essential oil drops in a diffuser.

2. Fill the diffuser with water according to the manufacturer's instructions.

3. Turn on the diffuser and enjoy the wonderful defense blend created in your space.

Note: This defense diffuser blend is not intended to treat or cure illnesses. It creates a refreshing and invigorating atmosphere in your home or office setting. Consult with a qualified aromatherapist or healthcare professional before using essential oils if you have any underlying health conditions, are pregnant, or are nursing.

∞ ∞ ∞

Skin Care and Beauty Recipes

Nourishing Facial Serum

A nourishing facial serum is essential to any skincare routine, and this product provides deep hydration and nourishment to the skin, improving health and appearance. The key to the serum's effectiveness lies in its carefully formulated composition.

With a high concentration of active ingredients, such as vitamins, antioxidants, and peptides, this powerhouse product delivers targeted benefits beyond what a regular moisturizer can offer. The vitamins present in the serum work to replenish and revitalize the skin, providing essential nutrients that promote a healthy complexion. Antioxidants help to combat the damaging effects of free radicals, which can contribute to premature aging and dullness.

By neutralizing these harmful molecules, antioxidants in the serum protect the skin from environmental stressors and promote a youthful glow. Peptides, known for their ability to stimulate collagen production, play a crucial role in restoring elasticity and firmness to the skin. They reduce the appearance of fine lines and wrinkles, resulting in a smooth and youthful complexion. Combining these powerful ingredients, a nourishing facial serum is a powerhouse product for the skin; therefore, by incorporating it into your skincare routine, you can achieve a radiant and healthy complexion that will make you feel confident and beautiful.

Improved Skin Hydration: is a nourishing facial serum designed to penetrate the skin and deliver essential nutrients and moisture to help effectively hydrate and moisturize the skin, leaving it plump, smooth, and glowing. This lightweight and easily absorbable formula of the serum makes it an ideal choice for those with dry skin.

Fine Lines and Wrinkles: Another benefit of using a nourishing facial serum is its ability to target visible signs of aging, such as fine lines and wrinkles. These serums have powerful anti-aging ingredients like retinol, peptides, and antioxidants, which help to stimulate collagen production and promote cell turnover. Therefore, using this serum would lead to a smoother, more youthful complexion with diminished signs of aging.

Brightened and Even Skin Tone: A nourishing facial serum can also contribute to a brighter and more even skin tone. Many serums contain ingredients like vitamin C and niacinamide, which work to fade dark spots, hyperpigmentation, and sun damage. Regular use of a serum results in a more radiant and uniform complexion, as well as improved overall skin texture.

Skin Firmness and Elasticity: As we age, our skin loses elasticity and starts to sag. However, a nourishing facial serum can help combat this issue. Serums that contain peptides and hyaluronic acid can improve skin firmness and elasticity, making it appear more lifted and toned. By replenishing the skin's natural moisture barrier and supporting collagen production, serums help improve the overall youthfulness and resilience of the skin.

Protection and Repair from Environmental Stressors: Our skin is constantly unprotected from environmental stressors such as pollution, UV radiation, and free radicals, which can cause damage and accelerate skin aging. A nourishing facial serum often contains antioxidants, like vitamin E and green tea extract, that help neutralize free radicals and protect the skin from oxidative stress. Additionally, serums with soothing ingredients can aid in the repair of existing damage and reduce inflammation.

In conclusion, incorporating a nourishing facial serum into your skincare routine can offer numerous benefits for your skin. From improved hydration and reduction in signs of aging to brighter skin tone and enhanced firmness, a serum provides targeted care and helps achieve a healthier and more youthful complexion. Additionally, serum protective and reparative properties make them valuable to any skincare regimen; so, if you want to rejuvenate your skin and maintain its health, a nourishing facial serum is undoubtedly worth considering for your skin is essential for maintaining a healthy and youthful complexion.

One way to give your skin a nourishing boost is by incorporating a facial serum into your skincare routine. When using a facial serum, it is essential to start with a clean and toned face; by removing any dirt or impurities, you ensure that the serum can penetrate the skin effectively. Once your face is ready, take a few drops of the serum onto your fingertips. The serum should feel lightweight and luxurious when applied to your skin. Use a gentle, upward circular motion to massage the serum into your face and neck.

This technique helps to stimulate blood flow and improves the absorption of the serum into your skin. Allow the serum to fully absorb before moving on to the next step. To lock in all the goodness of the serum, follow up with a moisturizer; by applying a moisturizer after the serum, you create a barrier that seals in the benefits and ensures that your skin stays hydrated throughout the day. Use a nourishing facial serum regularly; this will help improve the overall appearance and texture of the skin, leaving it looking radiant and rejuvenated. So why not give your skin the extra love and care it deserves by incorporating a nourishing facial serum into your skincare routine? When it comes to our skincare, it's crucial to understand that each person's skin is different from anyone else's, so we need to select a nourishing facial serum that should cater to your skin type with your specific concerns.

Different products target issues such as dryness, aging,

acne, or hyperpigmentation; therefore, choosing a specifically formulated serum for your skin's needs can enhance its overall health and appearance. However, it's essential to exercise caution when introducing a new skincare product to your routine. Our skin can sometimes react unexpectedly to certain ingredients, resulting in allergies or adverse reactions. For this reason, experts strongly recommend conducting a patch test before incorporating any new product into your regular skincare regimen. Patch testing involves applying a small amount of the product to a discreet area of your skin, such as behind your ear or on your inner arm, and observing any potential adverse effects. This precautionary step can help you identify any adverse reactions beforehand, allowing you to make informed decisions about the products you use and ensuring the best possible care for your unique skin.

Here is a recipe for a nourishing facial serum:

Ingredients:

- 1 tablespoon rosehip oil

- 1 tablespoon argan oil

- 1 tablespoon jojoba oil

- 5 drops of lavender essential oil

- 5 drops of frankincense essential oil

- 5 drops of geranium essential oil

Instructions:

1. combine the rosehip, argan, and jojoba oils in a small glass bottle.

2. Add the lavender, frankincense, and geranium essential oils to the mixture.

3. Seal the bottle tightly and shake well to blend all the ingredients.

4. After cleansing your face, apply a few drops of the serum onto your fingertips.

5. Gently massage the serum into your skin using upward circular motions until fully absorbed.

This nourishing facial serum has beneficial ingredients that moisturize and hydrate your skin while promoting a healthy complexion. Use it daily as part of your skincare routine for best results. Please note: Before using any new skincare product, it is advisable to perform a patch test to check for any potential allergic reactions or sensitivities.

Acne-Blasting Spot Treatment

Acne-blasting spot treatments have become a holy grail in skincare due to their ability to combat and eliminate those pesky acne spots or pimples. Acne products are to minimize the size, redness, and inflammation of every breakout; however, their incredible efficacy lies in their powerful active ingredients of benzoyl peroxide, salicylic acid, sulfur, or tea tree oil.

These superstar components work synergistically to penetrate the pores, eradicate harmful bacteria, and tame excessive oil production. By tackling the root causes of acne, these treatments bring immediate relief and prevent future breakouts, allowing individuals to regain their confidence and achieve a smooth and flawless complexion.

To use an acne-blasting spot treatment, follow these general steps:

1. Start with clean skin: Wash your face with a gentle cleanser and pat dry with a clean towel.

2. Apply the treatment: Using a clean fingertip or a cotton swab, apply a small amount of the spot treatment directly onto the acne spot or pimple. Avoid applying it to surrounding healthy skin.

3. Let it absorb: Allow the treatment to absorb fully into the skin. This usually takes a few minutes.

4. Follow with moisturizer: After the spot treatment has been absorbed, apply a light moisturizer to keep the skin hydrated.

5. Use as directed: Spot treatments can be applied once or twice daily, depending on the product instructions. It is essential to use these treatments sparingly as they can cause dryness and irritation.

When dealing with acne, it is crucial to understand the correct usage of spot treatments that treat individual acne spots rather than being applied to larger areas on the face. While spot treatments can effectively reduce the appearance of blemishes, using them all over your face or as a preventative measure may lead to skin dryness, irritation, or other unwanted side effects. It is vital to follow the instructions provided by the product and only apply it directly to the acne spot.

However, if your acne persists or worsens despite using spot treatments correctly, it is highly advisable to seek professional help. Consulting with a dermatologist is crucial at this stage. They possess the expertise to evaluate your skin condition and identify the underlying causes of your acne. A dermatologist will then be able to develop a customized treatment plan tailored to your specific needs, which could involve prescribing medication, suggesting lifestyle changes, or recommending other forms of treatment, such as skin-care routines or procedures. Seeking professional guidance ensures you receive targeted and effective solutions for your acne, ultimately leading to healthier skin.

Here is a recipe for an effective spot treatment to help combat acne:

Ingredients:

- 1 teaspoon tea tree oil

- 1 teaspoon witch hazel

- 1 teaspoon aloe vera gel

Instructions:

1. combine the tea tree oil, witch hazel, and aloe vera gel in a small bowl.

2. Mix well until all the ingredients are thoroughly blended.

3. Using a cotton swab or clean fingers, apply a small amount of the mixture directly onto the affected areas.

4. Leave it on overnight or for at least 30 minutes before rinsing off with water.

5. Repeat this process daily until you notice an improvement in your skin.

This homemade spot treatment combines the antibactcrial properties of tea tree oil with the soothing effects of witch hazel and aloe vera gel. It can help reduce inflammation and speed up the healing process of acne blemishes. Please note that all skin types are different, so it is important to patch test before applying this treatment to your whole face.

Radiant Hair Mask

Radiant Hair Mask is a luxurious and highly effective deep conditioning treatment that goes above and beyond to nourish and revitalize dry, damaged, or dull hair. This hair mask is a remarkable formula crafted with an exquisite blend of natural ingredients chosen for its exceptional moisturizing and repairing properties. Among these stellar ingredients, argan oil takes the lead, with its rich concentration of essential fatty acids and vitamin E.

This potent combination works wonders in restoring and rejuvenating your hair, leaving it unbelievably soft, silky, and lustrous. In addition to the benefits of argan oil, the Radiant Hair Mask also features the extraordinary moisturizing abilities of coconut oil. This tropical delight is famous for penetrating deep into the hair shaft, replenishing and hydrating even the most parched strands, resulting in a beautifully resilient and voluminous mane.

To further enhance the repairing power of this miraculous hair treatment, shea butter is expertly incorporated. Shea butter, derived from the nut of the African shea tree, boasts an impressive array of vitamins and antioxidants that diligently work to repair damage and prevent breakage, simultaneously providing an intense dose of hydration. The shea hair treatment's natural ingredients make Radiant Hair Mask a fantastic hair care treatment.

Say goodbye to lackluster and lifeless locks and say hello to a world of radiant, healthy hair. Whether you have chemically treated hair, heat-damaged strands, or a yearning for more vibrant hair, this deep conditioning treatment is your ultimate solution. Pamper yourself and indulge in the luxury of the Radiant Hair Mask for hair that exudes brilliance and vitality, giving you the confidence to conquer one fabulous hair day at a time.

The mask is a highly effective hair treatment that goes

beyond surface-level nourishment. It works its magic by deeply penetrating the hair shaft, delivering much-needed hydration to the core of each strand. This deep hydration not only moisturizes the hair but also works to restore its natural shine and softness. Dry and dull hair becomes a thing of the past as the mask works to revive and rejuvenate every strand, leaving it looking healthier and more vibrant.

In addition to its hydrating properties, the mask also has the added benefit of helping to detangle unruly strands. It works through knots and tangles, making combing or brushing a breeze. No more painful pulling or frustrating struggles with knotted hair; therefore, this detangling effect from the mask saves time but minimizes hair breakage and damage, allowing the hair to stay healthy and strong. Furthermore, this remarkable mask is a savior for those experiencing frizzy hair. With just a single use, it helps to reduce frizz, ultimately making the hair more manageable and more accessible to style. No longer will you have to battle with flyways or spend hours trying to tame your curly locks. The mask smooths down frizz and creates a more polished and put-together look, whether you wear your hair straight, curly, or in any other style.

In conclusion, the mask not only provides intense hydration to the hair but also offers a multitude of other benefits. From restoring natural shine and softness to aiding in detangling and reducing frizz, it transforms dull, unruly hair into a head of healthy, manageable, and lustrous locks. Say goodbye to bad hair days and embrace a newfound confidence in your hair's appearance and overall health with the help of this exceptional mask.

To effectively use the Radiant Hair Mask, it suggests that your hair is clean and towel-dried. Then, generously apply the mask to your hair, focusing on the mid-lengths to ends, where the hair tends to be drier and more damaged. The mask's rich and nourishing formula penetrates deeply into the hair fibers, delivering intense hydration and repairing any damage. Once applied, leave the hair mask on for approximately 5 to

10 minutes, allowing it ample time to work its magic. During this time, the mask's ingredients deeply penetrate the hair shaft, replenishing moisture and restoring vitality. For extra conditioning, you can cover your hair with a shower cap or wrap it in a warm towel, which helps to create a gentle heat, allowing the mask to penetrate the hair even further for a more intensive treatment. After the recommended treatment time, thoroughly rinse the mask with warm water and enjoy the luxurious feeling of silky, radiant hair. Consistently incorporating this hair mask into your hair care routine will leave you with healthier, more vibrant locks.

Once the recommended time for leaving the Radiant Hair Mask on your hair has elapsed, it is advisable to rinse your hair thoroughly and proceed to style it as per your usual routine. The unique formula of this hair mask has an instant effect, which can be observed immediately after rinsing. Your hair will feel noticeably smoother and softer and exude a radiant shine. However, the benefits of this hair mask extend beyond just one application.

Regularly using this Radiant Hair Mask can help enhance your hair's overall health and appearance. So, provide your hair with the nourishment and care it deserves by integrating this mask into your haircare routine to achieve your desired hair goals.

This recipe is for a hair mask that will leave your hair looking and feeling radiant. To make this mask, you will need the following:

Ingredients

- 1 ripe avocado

- 2 tablespoons of coconut oil

- 1 tablespoon of honey

- 1 tablespoon of apple cider vinegar

Start by mashing the avocado until it is smooth and creamy, then add the coconut oil, honey, and apple cider vinegar into the bowl and mix everything well. Once the mask is mixed, apply it to your hair from roots to ends, massaging it into your scalp. Leave this mask on for about 30 minutes to allow it to nourish deeply into the hair. After 30 minutes, rinse out this mask with warm water and follow with your regular shampoo and conditioner routine. You will immediately notice that your hair looks shinier and feels softer. Use this hair mask once a week for best results. Your locks will thank you!

∞ ∞ ∞

Household Cleaning Recipes

Natural All-Purpose Cleaner

A natural all-purpose cleaner is an effective cleaning product but a safer option for your home. Conventional cleaners that contain harmful chemicals, a natural all-purpose cleaner is made with natural ingredients that arc non-toxic and environmentally friendly. That means you can use it to clean different surfaces in your home without worrying about exposing yourself or your loved ones to harmful substances.

The beauty of a natural all-purpose cleaner lies in its versatility. With just a few simple ingredients, you can create a cleaner that you can use on many surfaces, including kitchen countertops, bathroom tiles, windows, mirrors, and much more. That saves you from buying multiple cleaning products and simplifies your cleaning routine.

One of the most popular recipes for a natural all-purpose cleaner involves mixing equal parts of white vinegar and water. Vinegar is a natural disinfectant that can effectively kill germs and bacteria, making it an excellent choice for cleaning and sanitizing surfaces. Additionally, it helps to remove tough stains and odors. When combined with water, it creates a mild yet powerful solution that can tackle dirt and grime without leaving behind residue or chemical fumes.

When using a natural all-purpose cleaner, add a pleasant fragrance with a few drops of essential oils with some common choices, including lavender, lemon, orange, and tea tree oil. Not only do these oils leave behind a refreshing scent, but they also have natural antibacterial properties that further boost the cleaning power of your homemade cleaner.

With a natural all-purpose cleaner, you can achieve a sparkling clean home while minimizing your environmental impact and protecting your health. It's a win-win situation, allowing you to maintain a clean and healthy living space without compromising your values. So why not make your natural all-purpose cleaner today?

Ingredients:

- 1 cup of distilled water

- 1 cup of white vinegar

- 10-15 drops of essential oil (such as lemon, lavender, orange, or tea tree

Instructions:

1. Mix the distilled water and white vinegar in a spray bottle.

2. Add the essential oil of your choice to the mixture.

3. Close the spray bottle and shake well to combine all the ingredients.

The natural all-purpose cleaner is a versatile and effective cleaning solution. It offers a convenient way to maintain cleanliness throughout your home. This spray can disinfect and refresh surfaces such as countertops, appliances, bathroom fixtures, and glass. Its multi-purpose formula makes it suitable for tackling different types of grime and dirt. Whether it's a spilled drink on the kitchen counter, a fingerprint on the fridge, soap scum on the shower fixtures, or streaks on the windows, this cleaner is up to the task. After spraying, you can effortlessly wipe away the mess with a microfiber cloth or sponge, leaving the surfaces sparkling clean and clear of residue. Using this natural all-purpose cleaner, you can confidently maintain a hygienic and fresh environment within your home without the need for harmful chemicals.

The white vinegar in the cleaner plays a vital role in

maintaining a clean and healthy environment. Not only does it effectively disinfect surfaces, but it also performs admirably in stain removal. Its natural properties allow it to combat stubborn stains and break them down, leaving surfaces fresh and spotless. In addition to its cleaning power, white vinegar complements essential oil in the cleaner. This aromatic addition not only provides a pleasant and refreshing scent but may also contribute to the eradication of harmful microorganisms. With potential antimicrobial properties, the essential oil ensures a clean and hygienic surface. To guarantee purity, distilled water is added to the formula through a purification process to eliminate any impurities that could mar the cleanliness of surfaces and leave unsightly streaks or residues.

When it comes to cleaning, it's always best to be cautious. No matter how effective a cleaner may claim to be, it's essential to test it out on a small, inconspicuous area first. This simple step can save you from trouble and prevent damage on a larger surface, whereas doing a compatibility test will determine if the cleaner is suitable for the material. However, many cleaning surfaces require different cleaning solutions to achieve optimal results. So, before you embark on your cleaning spree, take a moment to protect your furniture, carpets, or any other surfaces by performing a patch test. This small act of precaution can go a long way in maintaining the integrity and longevity of your belongings.

Sparkling Dishwasher Tabs

A natural all-purpose cleaner is an effective cleaning product but a safer option for your home. Unlike conventional cleaners that have harmful chemicals, a natural all-purpose cleaner made with natural ingredients is non-toxic and environmentally friendly. With that said, you can use it to clean different surfaces in your home without worrying about exposing yourself or your loved ones to harmful substances.

The beauty of a natural all-purpose cleaner lies in its

versatility. This cleaner can be used on many surfaces, including kitchen countertops, bathroom tiles, windows, mirrors, and more, when combining simple ingredients. This cleaner will save you from buying multiple cleaning products and simplifies your cleaning routine.

One of the most popular recipes for a natural all-purpose cleaner involves mixing equal parts of white vinegar and water. Vinegar is a natural disinfectant that can effectively kill germs and bacteria, making it an excellent choice for cleaning and sanitizing surfaces. Additionally, it helps to remove tough stains and odors. When combined with water, it creates a mild yet powerful solution that can tackle dirt and grime without leaving behind residue or chemical fumes.

When enhancing the natural all-purpose cleaning properties, add a pleasant fragrance to your cleaner by including a few drops of essential oils. Common choices include lavender, lemon, orange, and tea tree oil. Not only do these oils leave behind a refreshing scent, but they also have natural antibacterial properties that further boost the cleaning power of your homemade cleaner.

With a natural all-purpose cleaner, you can achieve a sparkling clean home while minimizing your environmental impact and protecting your health. It's a win-win situation by allowing you to maintain a clean and healthy living space without compromising your values. So, give it a try and make your natural all-purpose cleaner today.

Ingredients:

- 1 cup of distilled water

- 1 cup of white vinegar

- 10-15 drops of essential oil (such as lemon, lavender, orange, or tea tree

Instructions:

1. Mix the distilled water and white vinegar in a spray bottle.

2. Add the essential oil of your choice to the mixture.

3. Close the spray bottle and shake well to combine all the ingredients.

The natural all-purpose cleaner is a versatile and effective cleaning solution. It offers a convenient way to maintain cleanliness throughout your home. A simple cleaner spray can disinfect and refresh surfaces such as countertops, appliances, bathroom fixtures, and glass. Its multi-purpose formula makes it suitable for tackling different types of grime and dirt. Whether it's a spilled drink on the kitchen counter, a fingerprint on the fridge, soap scum on the shower fixtures, or streaks on the windows, this cleaner is up to the task. After spraying, you can effortlessly wipe away the mess with a microfiber cloth or sponge, leaving the surfaces sparkling clean and clear of residue. Using this natural all-purpose cleaner, you can confidently maintain a hygienic and fresh environment within your home without the need for harmful chemicals.

The white vinegar in the cleaner plays a vital role in

maintaining a clean and healthy environment. Not only does it effectively disinfect surfaces, but it also performs admirably in stain removal. Its natural properties allow it to combat stubborn stains and break them down, leaving surfaces fresh and spotless. In addition to its cleaning power, white vinegar complements the inclusion of essential oil in the cleaner. This aromatic addition not only provides a pleasant and refreshing scent but may also contribute to the eradication of harmful microorganisms. With potential antimicrobial properties, the essential oil ensures a clean and hygienic surface. When adding distilled water to the cleaner's formula, the water undergoes a purification process that decreases impurities that could mar the cleanliness of surfaces and leave unsightly streaks or residues, giving peace of mind with the knowledge of having pristine surfaces.

When it comes to cleaning, it's always best to be cautious. No matter how effective a cleaner may claim to be, it's essential to test it out on a small, inconspicuous area first. This simple step can save you from trouble and prevent damage on a larger surface by doing a compatibility test to determine if the cleaner is reliable for the material. Many characters have different requirements for cleaning solutions, and it is crucial to choose the right one to achieve optimal results. So, before you embark on your cleaning spree, take a moment to protect your furniture, carpets, or any other surfaces by performing a patch test. This small act of precaution can go a long way in maintaining the integrity and longevity of your belongings.

Fresh Linen Spray

Fresh Linen spray is essential to revitalize and impart a delightful, clean fragrance to various items in our homes. This remarkable product works wonders on clothing, linens, and upholstery, transforming them from dull and lifeless to refreshed and invigorated. The convenient spray bottle packaging ensures ease of use, allowing one to effortlessly apply it onto the desired fabric or disperse it into the air, dispelling any unpleasant odors and infusing the surroundings with a crisp and revitalizing aroma. Whether it is eliminating the lingering smell of smoke or simply enhancing the overall ambiance of a room, Fresh Linen spray never fails to deliver outstanding results. Combining versatility and effectiveness, it has become an indispensable tool in our cleaning routines and a dependable solution for maintaining a pleasant and inviting atmosphere within our homes. Some scents for fresh linen sprays include:

Lavender: Known for its calming and relaxing properties, lavender-scented linen spray is a soothing ambiance in bedrooms and living spaces.

Citrus: Citrus-scented linen sprays, such as lemon or orange, are refreshing and invigorating. They are often used in kitchens or bathrooms to eliminate cooking or bathroom odors.

Eucalyptus: Eucalyptus-scented linen sprays are known for their fresh and energizing aroma. They are often used in laundry rooms to add a clean scent to freshly washed clothes.

Fresh Cotton: A popular fresh cotton-scented linen spray that smells like freshly laundered clothes and gives a clean and crisp aroma to linen and upholstery.

Ocean Breeze: Ocean breeze-scented linen sprays provide a fresh and cool aroma reminiscent of the sea. They are often used in bathrooms or bedrooms to create a relaxing and refreshing atmosphere.

The fresh linen spray is a simple and effective way to refresh your fabrics. First, to make the most of this product, give a good shake to the bottle, which will help to mix the ingredients and ensure the scent has an even distribution; therefore, place the bottle a few inches away from the fabric and begin spraying in a sweeping motion evenly coating the material. Next, this linen spray on the fabric, allowing time to dry, will help the scent absorb without transferring or staining other surfaces. The scent duration will vary depending on the brand of linen spray you are using. Some brands offer scents that last several hours or longer, allowing you to enjoy the refreshing fragrance for an extended period. Overall, using fresh linen spray is a convenient way to revive and enhance the scent of your fabrics.

Here is a recipe for fresh linen spray:

Ingredients:

- 1 cup distilled water

- 2 tablespoons vodka or rubbing alcohol

- 10 drops of lavender essential oil

- 5 drops of lemon essential oil

- 5 drops of eucalyptus essential oil

Instructions:

1. In a small spray bottle, combine the distilled water and vodka or rubbing alcohol.

2. Add the lavender, lemon, and eucalyptus essential oils to the bottle.

3. Close the bottle and shake well to mix all the ingredients.

4. To use, spray your freshly washed linens before putting them away or onto pillows and sheets for a refreshing scent.

This homemade fresh linen spray is a great way to add a pleasant aroma to your linens while providing relaxation benefits from the soothing scents of lavender, lemon, and eucalyptus. Enjoy!

Aromatic Remedies

Soothing Muscle Salve

A soothing muscle salve is a product specifically formulated to offer comfort and relaxation to tired, achy muscles. This topical ointment or balm has an ingredient combination with analgesic properties, such as menthol, camphor, or capsaicin. These components work together to create a numbing effect that helps temporarily alleviate any discomfort or pain one may be experiencing in their muscles. When applied to the skin, the soothing salve penetrates deeply, targeting the affected area and providing a calming sensation. By using a muscle salve regularly, individuals can benefit from the relief it provides, allowing them to relax and recover from their muscle-related discomfort.

A soothing muscle salve for pain and discomfort causing muscle soreness or strain where these types of salves often contain a combination of pain-relieving ingredients to alleviate the discomfort. These ingredients may include menthol, camphor, or lidocaine, which numbs the area and provides a cooling sensation that helps to dull the pain. However, a good muscle salve goes beyond just pain relief. It may also incorporate ingredients with anti-inflammatory properties to further reduce swelling and inflammation in the muscles. Some common examples are arnica and turmeric, both known for their natural anti-inflammatory effects. Including these ingredients in the salve can help improve healing and accelerate recovery. Soothing muscle salves can be a valuable addition to any first aid kit or wellness routine, as they provide targeted relief for specific muscle-related discomfort and promote a faster and more comfortable recovery.

In addition to essential oils like lavender or eucalyptus, muscle salves often contain other common ingredients that contribute to their effectiveness. These ingredients may include menthol, which creates a cooling sensation on the skin and helps relieve muscle soreness or discomfort. Another common addition is arnica, a natural herb that reduces inflammation and bruising. However, ingredients like camphor or wintergreen oil are known for their analgesic properties, which provide pain relief. These additional essential oil ingredients create a powerful and soothing balm for tired or achy muscles.

Using a soothing muscle salve is an effective way to alleviate discomfort and promote overall muscle relaxation. It is a simple process that involves applying a small amount of muscle salve onto the affected area and gently massaging it into the skin. After application, the active ingredients in the muscle salve work together to target the source of pain, reducing its intensity and providing much-needed relief. The gentle massage also enhances the absorption of the muscle salve, allowing the muscles to benefit fully from its soothing properties.

As the salve begins to take effect, a calming sensation emerges, melting away tension and easing the stiffness in the muscles. Therefore, this promotes relaxation and rejuvenation throughout the body, enabling you to move freely without discomfort. When experiencing muscle soreness from intense physical activity or dealing with muscle tension due to stress, add this muscle salve to your self-care routine; by incorporating this natural and comforting remedy into your daily routine, you can experience the soothing benefits it has to offer and enjoy a greater sense of ease and well-being.

When dealing with muscle soreness, it is crucial to understand that a soothing muscle salve can only offer temporary relief. While it may alleviate discomfort for a short period, it is essential to remember that it should not be a substitute for proper medical care. In cases where you are facing chronic or severe muscle pain, always seek guidance from a certified healthcare professional. They possess the knowledge and expertise to provide you with an accurate diagnosis and develop an appropriate treatment plan tailored specifically to your needs. When consulting with a healthcare professional, address the condition and the underlying cause for the muscle pain, resulting in long-term relief and improved well-being.

Here is a recipe for a soothing muscle salve:

Ingredients:

- 1 cup of coconut oil

- 1/4 cup of beeswax pellets

- 20 drops of peppermint essential oil

- 15 drops of lavender essential oil

- 10 drops of eucalyptus essential oil

Instructions:

1. In a double boiler, melt the coconut oil and beeswax pellets together until thoroughly melted and combined.

2. Remove from heat and let it cool slightly.

3. Add the peppermint, lavender, and eucalyptus essential oils to the mixture and stir well.

4. Pour the mixture into small containers or tins and let it cool completely before sealing.

Apply a small amount of the soothing muscle salve to the skin and massage gently onto sore muscles or joints. Therefore, this muscle salve will offer relief and relaxation after physical activity or for general muscle discomfort. Please note that it's always advisable to perform a patch test before using any new product on your skin if you have known allergies or sensitivities. If any irritation occurs, discontinue use immediately.

Earache Relief Oil

Earache relief oil is a popular choice for those seeking a natural solution to alleviate the pain and discomfort caused by earaches. The relief oil has ingredients from garlic, mullein, or tea tree oil, which have anti-inflammatory properties and combat infections. Garlic has potent antibacterial and antiviral properties to help effectively fight off underlying impurities that may contribute to earaches.

Mullein possesses soothing and analgesic qualities that provide much-needed relief from the pain associated with earaches. Tea tree oil is renowned for its antimicrobial properties, which help reduce inflammation and prevent infection. By combining these beneficial ingredients, earache relief oils offer a holistic approach to managing the symptoms of earaches without resorting to harsh chemicals or medications. Moreover, these natural remedies are easy to use and can be applied externally, providing almost immediate relief. Whether the earache is from an infection, congestion, or simply due to the discomfort of wax build-up, earache relief oils are a gentle and effective option for soothing the pain and promoting quick healing.

Garlic oil: Garlic has natural antibiotic and anti-inflammatory properties, which may help fight infection and reduce pain. Therefore, the cloves are crushed and infused with olive or almond oil to prepare the garlic oil.

Mullein oil: Mullein has soothing properties for relieving ear pain and inflammation. Mullein oil can be made by steeping the dried leaves and flowers of the mullein plant in a carrier oil.

Tea tree oil: Tea tree oil has antiseptic and antimicrobial properties, which may help combat infections that cause earaches. Tea tree oil is diluted with a carrier oil and applied topically around the outside of the ear.

When finding relief for any medical condition, including ear pain, it is crucial to prioritize one's health and safety. While essential oils have gained popularity for their potential therapeutic benefits, it is important to remember that they should never be a replacement for professional medical treatment. With the use of essential oils, it should be a complementary approach to managing symptoms rather than a standalone solution. In cases of severe or persistent ear pain, seeking the guidance and expertise of a healthcare professional is highly recommended.

They possess the knowledge and training necessary to accurately diagnose the underlying cause of the pain and provide proper treatment. Consulting with a healthcare professional ensures that one receives appropriate medical care tailored to specific conditions, potentially preventing further complications or issues that arise from solely relying on self-treatment methods. Therefore, it is necessary to exercise caution and responsibility when dealing with any health concern and be proactive in seeking the appropriate care to address the root cause of the problem.

Here is a recipe for an earache relief oil:

Ingredients:

- 2 tablespoons of olive oil

- 5 drops of lavender essential oil

- 3 drops of tea tree essential oil

- 2 drops of chamomile essential oil

- 1 drop of peppermint essential oil

Instructions:

1. In a small bowl, combine the olive oil with the essential oils.

2. Mix well until all the ingredients are evenly combined.

3. carefully transfer the mixture into a small glass bottle

using a dropper.

4. Ensure that the bottle is tightly sealed to preserve the freshness and potency of the oils.

5. To use, warm a few drops of the earache relief oil by rubbing it between your palms.

6. Gently massage the warm oil onto and around your earlobe, avoiding contact with your eardrum.

7. Repeat this process as needed for soothing relief from ear pain.

Note: Please consult a healthcare professional before using homemade remedies, especially if you have severe or persistent ear pain.

This homemade earache relief oil can be a natural and gentle option for alleviating earache discomfort. Combining olive oil and essential oils such as lavender, tea tree, chamomile, and peppermint can provide soothing properties that may help ease inflammation and reduce pain in the affected area. However, it's important to remember that each person's sensitivity to essential oils may vary, so perform a patch test before applying to ensure no adverse reactions.

Additionally, if symptoms persist or worsen over time, seek medical advice from a healthcare professional for proper diagnosis and treatment options. Remember to store this DIY earache relief oil in a cool, dark place to maintain its effectiveness for future use. Note: Please consult a healthcare professional before using homemade remedies, especially if you have severe or persistent ear pain.

Sinus Congestion Inhalation Blend

Sinus congestion inhalation blends are a popular remedy when individuals suffer from respiratory issues. These blends are combined using essential oils known for their powerful decongestant, anti-inflammatory, and antimicrobial properties. Therefore, essential oil blends alleviate sinus congestion and promote easier breathing.

When sinus congestion strikes, it can be incredibly uncomfortable, making breathing difficult and causing pain in the head and face. Using inhalation blends will decrease an individual's symptoms and allow them to find greater comfort.

The essential oils have decongestant properties to help clear the nasal passages and reduce the inflammation that often accompanies sinus congestion. Therefore, it provides immediate relief and promotes long-term healing by addressing the underlying cause of the congestion. Moreover, the oil's anti-inflammatory properties help reduce swelling in the sinus cavities, allowing for airflow and improved respiratory function. Inflammation is a common culprit in sinus congestion, and by combating it with natural remedies, individuals can find relief without resorting to over-the-counter medications.

The antimicrobial properties in essential oils help to combat any potential infections that may be causing or exacerbating sinus congestion. These oils have shown powerful antibacterial and antiviral effects, helping to eliminate harmful pathogens and boost the immune system.

Sinus congestion inhalation blends offer a natural and effective solution for individuals seeking relief from respiratory issues. By harnessing the power of essential oils, these blends relieve congestion, promote easier breathing, and support overall respiratory health due to allergies, colds, or other sinus-related issues. The oil blends are valuable for managing symptoms and wellness.

Here is a simple inhalation blend recipe:

Ingredients:

- 2 drops eucalyptus essential oil

- 2 drops peppermint essential oil

- 2 drops of tea tree essential oil

- 1 drop of lavender essential oil

- 1 drop of rosemary essential oil

Instructions:

1. Fill a small amber glass bottle with a roller top or dropper with the essential oils.

2. Close the bottle and gently shake it to mix the oils.

3. To use, roll the blend onto your palms and cup your hands over your nose and mouth, taking deep breaths in through your nose and out through your mouth.

4. Add a few drops of the blend to a diffuser or a bowl of hot water and inhale the steam.

5. Store the inhalation blend in a cool, dark place when not in use.

When using essential oils, it is crucial to exercise caution; however, these oils are highly concentrated and should be used with care when applied to the skin or inhaled. Though essential oils have been around for centuries and are valuable, they may not be suitable for anyone with underlying medical conditions. Before incorporating essential oils into your wellness routine, you must consult a healthcare professional. Similarly, if you are pregnant or breastfeeding, seek guidance from a healthcare professional, as certain essential oils may not be safe during these stages. By taking these precautions, you can ensure that your experience with essential oils is positive and safe.

In conclusion, Aromatherapy & Essential Oils open up a whole new realm of possibilities as they bring you into the fascinating world of essential oils. This book emphasized the importance of caution when using these concentrated substances, reminding readers to perform a patch test and consult a professional if they have any concerns or medical conditions. Therefore, fear not, for within the pages of this book lies a plethora of remedies to fulfill your desires for relaxation, rejuvenation, or simply a little natural support. So, even if you are a beginner to aromatherapy and essential oils, this will make it easier to follow along and create your blends. So, dive into nature, surround yourself with incredible aromas, and embark on this delightful and transformative journey. Your senses will thank you as you indulge in the wonders of aromatherapy.

∞ ∞ ∞

Favorite Recipes

Homemade Makeup Remover

Ingredients:
- 4 Tbsp of Witch Hazel
- 2 Tbsp of pure Jojoba Oil
- 2 Tbsp of Extra Virgin Olive Oil
- 3 Tbsp of Purified Water

Instructions:
1. Use a small glass bottle or jar.
2. Start by putting the Witch Hazel into the container.
3. Add the Jojoba and Olive Oil.
4. Add the water to the container, place the lid on it, and shake it to blend well.
5. To use, shake the container each time before application. Then, use a cotton ball or pad and wipe the face gently using the makeup remover until all makeup is removed.

Lavender and Rose Water Toner

Ingredients:
- 4 Tbsp of Rose Water
- 2 Tbsp of Witch Hazel
- 1 tsp of Apple Cider Vinegar
- 5-10 drops of Rosehip Oil
- Five drops of Tea Tree Oil
- Five drops of Lavender Oil or your favorite essential oil scent.

Instructions:
1. Get a small bowl and whisk or spoon.
2. Start by putting Rosehip Water, Witch Hazel, Apple Cider Vinegar, Rosehip Oil, Tea Tree Oil, and Lavender into the bowl.
3. Transfer to a small glass spray bottle.
4. Add the water to the container, place the lid on it, and shake it to blend well.
5. To use, cleanse the face well, close your eyes, and spray the toner onto the face.
6. Add your favorite natural facial moisturizer.

Calming Body Butter

Ingredients:
- ¼ cup of Avocado Oil
- ¼ cup of Magnesium Oil
- ¾ cup of Cocoa Butter
- 30 drops of Lavender Oil

Instructions:
1. Use a large glass jar.
2. Place water in a saucepan over low heat, place the container with the Cocoa Butter.
3. Once melted, pour into a bowl and let cool in the fridge for 30 minutes.
4. I am using a standard mixer blend and whip it.
5. Once mixed, add in Magnesium Oil, Avocado Oil, and essential oils and mix
6. Transfer to the glass jar or plastic container and keep in the refrigerator for 90 days.

Body Butter Lotion

Ingredients:
- ½ cup of Shea Butter
- 1/8 cup of Jojoba Oil
- ½ cup of Coconut Oil
- 20 drops of Essential Oil (Choose your favorite scent)

Instructions:
1. Place a saucepan filled with water on the stove on medium heat.
2. Place in a glass bowl with Shea Butter, Coconut Oil, and Jojoba Oil into the saucepan.
3. Once melted, mix, then put into the refrigerator for an hour or until solid.
4. With a hand mixer, beat the oils until they are whipped and fluffy
5. Mix in your favorite essential oils
6. Fill a container with the body butter mixture and store it at room temperature.

Face wash

Ingredients:
- 1 cup of Coconut Oil
- 1 Tbsp of Baking Soda
- Five drops of Lavender essential oil
- Five drops of Frankincense essential oil
- Five drops of Lemon essential oil
- If acne-prone, replace Frankincense and Lemon oils with ten drops of Tea Tree essential oil.

Instructions:
1. Use a glass jar.
2. Melt the Coconut oil in a pan over low heat.
3. Once melted, remove from heat and add in remaining ingredients.
4. Store in a wash dispenser or air-tight jar, and keep it in a cool place.

Homemade Body Wash

Ingredients:
- 1 cup of Water
- ¼ cup of Honey
- 2/3 cup of Liquid Castille Soap
- 30 drops of Lavender Oil, Chamomile, or Geranium Essential Oils
- 1 tsp of Jojoba Oil

Instructions:
1. BPA-free plastic lotion dispenser or Glass bottle with dispenser.
2. Mix ingredients until smooth and store.

Coconut Lavender Shampoo

Ingredients:
- 1 ½ cups (1 can) of Coconut Milk
- 1 ½ cups of Liquid Castille Soap
- 40 drops of Lavender Essential Oil

Instructions:
1. BPA-free plastic dispenser bottle.
2. Mix well all ingredients in a bowl.
3. Pour mixture into a bottle.
4. Shake the bottle before each use.

Eye Cream

Ingredients:
- Ten drops of Frankincense Essential Oil
- 1 oz of Pure Aloe Vera Gel
- 1 oz of Unrefined Shea Butter
- 1 oz of Unrefined Coconut Oil
- ½ tsp of Vitamin E

Instructions:
1. In a small bowl, mix all the ingredients.
2. If needed, (during colder months warm) coconut oil and shea butter in a small pan.
3. Add the rest of the ingredients.
4. When well blended, transfer to a glass jar (if warmed up, let cool down first).
5. Use every morning and night around the eyes.

Anti-aging Serum

Ingredients:
- ½ Tbsp of Jojoba Oil
- ½ Tbsp of Evening Primrose Oil
- ½ Tbsp of Pomegranate Oil
- 15 drops of Vitamin E
- 20 drops of Lavender or Frankincense Oil
- Ten drops of Carrot Seed Oil

Instructions:
1. Mix all of the ingredients in a dark glass bottle.
2. Use every morning and night on the face, neck, and chest.

Morning Eye Solution

Ingredients:
- ½ oz Witch Hazel Extract
- Ten drops of Chamomile Essential Oil
- ½ oz of Pure Aloe Vera Gel
- Ten drops of Lavender Essential Oil

Instructions:
1. Combine all ingredients in a small glass jar with a lid.
2. Blend well.
3. Place into the refrigerator overnight.
4. Upon waking, apply a small amount of the solution around the eyes and let it sit as long as possible. Gently remove.
5. Apply a natural moisturizer.

Shaving Cream

Ingredients:
-   1/3 cup of Shea Butter
-   1/3 cup of Coconut Oil
-   ¼ cup of Jojoba Oil, Sweet Almond Oil, or Grapeseed Oil
-   Ten drops of Rosemary Essential Oil (For Men: Sandalwood Essential Oil and Cedarwood Essential Oil)
-   3-5 drops of Peppermint Oil

Instructions:
1. In a small saucepan over low heat, combine shea butter and coconut oil and stir until melted.
2. Transfer to a heat-safe bowl, add jojoba oil and essential oils.
3. Place the bowl into the refrigerator and chill until solid.
4. Remove from refrigerator, and use a mixer to whip until light and fluffy.
5. Spoon into a jar with a lid.
6. Keep in a cool, dry place.

Beard Oil

Ingredients:
- ½ oz of Jojoba Oil
- ½ oz of Sweet Almond Oil or Grapeseed Oil
- 1 Tbsp of Coconut Oil
- 3-4 drops of Cedarwood Essential Oil
- 3-4 drops of Sandalwood Essential Oil

Instructions:
1. In a small bottle with an eyedropper and cap, add jojoba oil.
2. Add sweet almond or grapeseed oil and coconut oil.
3. Add the cedarwood and sandalwood essential oils.
4. Place the top on tightly and shake well.
5. Using your hands or eyedropper, apply a few drops and massage into the beard and onto the cheeks.
6. Brush the beard for the finishing touches.

Allergy & Cold Remedy

Ingredients:
- Three large Lemons (Freshly squeezed or Lemon Juice)
- ¼ cup of Local Honey
- 3 Tbsp of Coconut Oil
- 1 tsp of Ground Cloves
- Ten drops of Lemon Essential Oil
- Three drops of Thieves Essential Oil

Instructions:
1. Heat all ingredients over medium heat and bring to a boil.
2. Then simmer on low heat for 20 minutes.
3. Cool for 20-30 minutes.
4. Store in a glass jar.
5. Take as needed.

Laundry Soap

Ingredients:
- 1 Box (65 oz) 20 Mule Team Borax
- 1 Box (55 oz) Arm & Hammer Super Wash
- 1 Box (4 lbs.) Baking Soda
- 1 Large Container (39 oz) Purex Crystals
- 1 Box (17.6 oz) Zote Soap
- 1 Container (1.77 lbs.) Oxy Clean
- 30 drops of Lavender Essential Oils

Instructions:
1. Mix all ingredients in a bucket.
2. Transfer ingredients into a container you would like to store your soap in.
3. Use one scoop (2-3 Tbsp) for each load of laundry.